Bong
Appétit

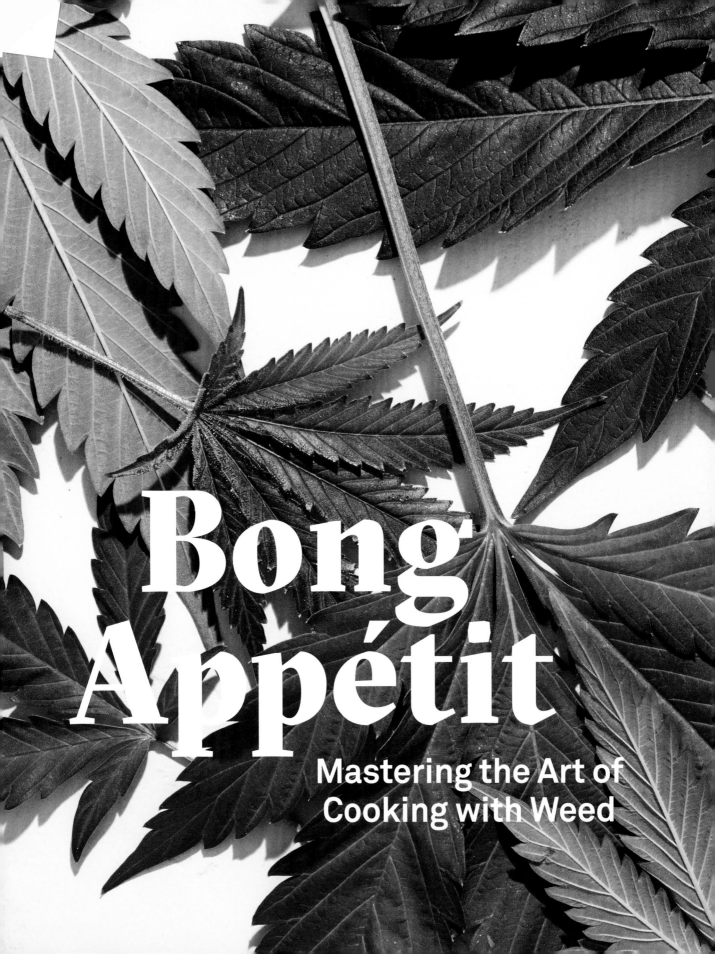

Bong Appétit

Mastering the Art of Cooking with Weed

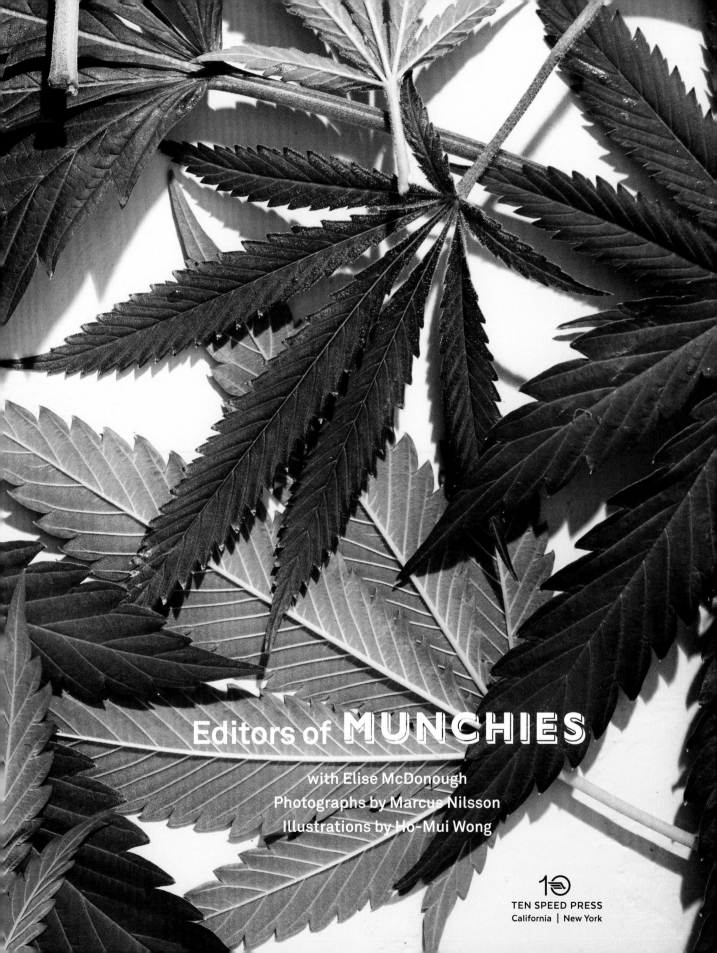

Editors of **MUNCHIES**

with Elise McDonough
Photographs by Marcus Nilsson
Illustrations by Ho-Mui Wong

TEN SPEED PRESS
California | New York

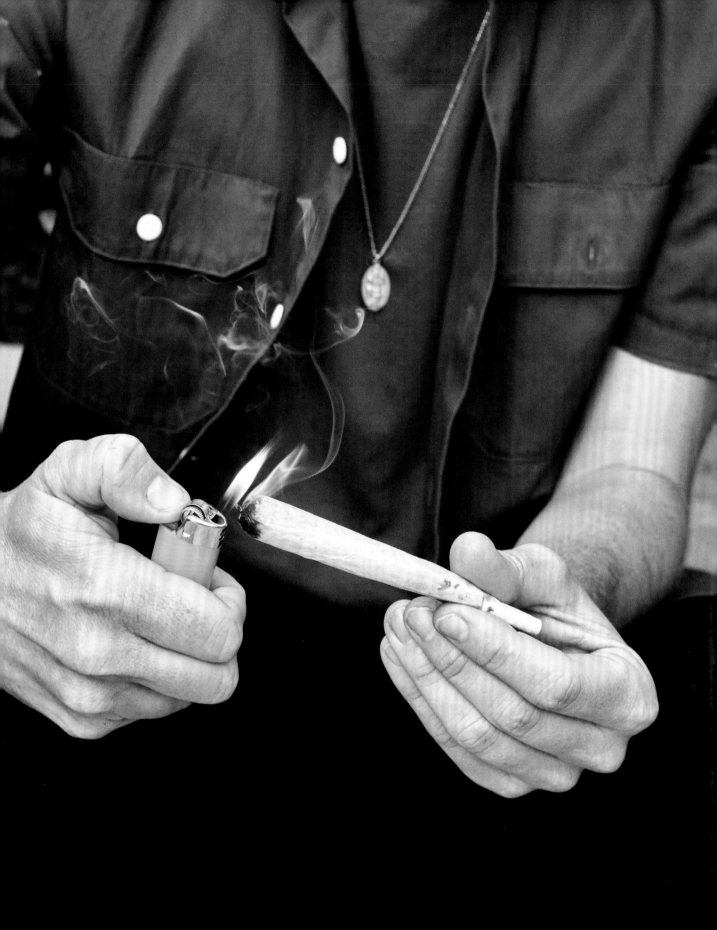

Contents

8 Introduction

61 Infusions

85 Drinks

97 Appetizers

117 Salads & Vegetables

139 Pasta & Grains

155 Meat, Poultry & Seafood

187 Desserts

217 Projects

246 Resources

249 Acknowledgments

252 Index

Infusions

Weed-Infused Oil 64

Weed-Infused Butter 68

Weed-Infused
   Brown Butter 70

Weed-Infused
   Coconut Milk 71

Weed-Infused Cream 72

Whipped Weed-Infused Honey
   or Syrup 74

Nitrous Green Dragon 77

Everclear Cannabis
   Tincture 80

Glycerin Cannabis Tincture 83

Drinks

Manhattan 87

Dirty Martini 87

White Negroni 88

French 75 90

Sangria 91

Margarita 93

Apple Bong 94

Appetizers

Sour Cream and Onion
   Nachos 99

Red Beet Pakoras 100

Sweet Potato Skins with
   Pancetta and Chipotle
   Crema 103

Fried Spring Rolls 105

Pork Wontons 108

French Bread Pizza 110

Blackened Shrimp
   Cocktail 113

Coconut Crab Gratin 114

Salads & Vegetables

Cucumber and Citrus
   Salad 119

Summer Tomato and
   Stone Fruit Salad 120

BLAT Salad 123

Creamy Cilantro Kale Salad
   with Coconut Bacon 124

North African Broccoli
   Salad 127

Hasselback Potatoes 129

Roasted Vegetables with
   Whipped Weed-Infused
   Honey 130

Fried Mixed Mushrooms 133

The Collard Green Melt 135

Pasta & Grains

Brown Butter Gnocchi 141

Green Mac and Cheese 145

Peanut Butter Noodles 146

Sausage Pappardelle
   Bolognese 149

Spinach and Artichoke Dip
   Risotto 150

Chicken Rice (Riz a Djaj) 152

Meat, Poultry & Seafood

Rib-Eye with Weed Chimichurri 157
Braised Short Ribs 158
"Sugaree" Pork Ribs 161
Yogurt-Marinated Lamb 162
Double-Lemon Roast Chicken 165
Korean Fried Chicken 166
Pakalolo Poke Bowl 169
Swordfish Teriyaki 170
Grilled Whole Sea Bream 173
Grilled Oysters 174
Fried Soft-Shell Crab with Shishito Pepper Mole 177
Green Shellfish Curry 180
Coconut Seafood Stew (Moqueca) 183
Confit Octopus 184

Desserts

Truffles 189
Stoner Candy Bites 190
Frozen Cocoa Pudding Pops 192
Honey Rosemary Ice Cream 193
Brownie Sundae 195
Salted Chocolate Chip Cookies 196
Raspberry and Peach Pie 198
Strawberry Shortcake Trifle 201
Strawberry "Cheesecake" 205
Bananas Foster 206
After-Dinner Mint Gummies 208
Adult Celebration Cake 211

Projects

Cannabis Leaf Pesto 219
Cannabis Leaf Chips 220
Herb Focaccia 223
Dinner Rolls 224
Corn Biscuits 226
Preserved Lemons 228
Cherry Elderberry Jam 230
Homemade Peanut Butter 232
Homemade Ricotta Cheese 233
Cannabis Kimchi 234
Gravlax 237
Pot Pepperoni 239
Hot or Sweet Italian Sausage 241
Broccoli Rabe and Provolone Sausage 244

Recipe List

Introduction

People have been eating weed for thousands of years—brewed for tea, crumbled into coffee, as a tincture, mixed with fruits and spice in jam—but in the last decade or so, it has started to feel very different. Building on the accumulated wisdom of traditional recipes such as Middle Eastern *mahjoun* and Indian *bhang,* cannabis cuisine has gone far beyond brownies and has reclaimed its place as a serious culinary ingredient. We're now living in a new era of marijuana cuisine; one of space-age vaporizers, designer hash, and cutting-edge science, all of which have helped take weed food to a whole other realm.

In these pages, we're experimenting with weed, but not like teenage stoners hitting a homemade gravity bong. Instead, we have enlisted some incredible chefs to make weed food that eclipses those early brownies—the kind of fare that you'd want to sit down and eat even if there wasn't weed in it.

Through a mash-up of modern cooking techniques and hard-won weed wisdom, television series *Bong Appétit* highlights next-level ingredients and techniques that are revolutionizing the way we use cannabis, as a culinary ingredient—leafy green; spice; dried herb; refined, isolated chemical—and as something that gets you high.

Envied for its extensive pantry filled with fine flowers, rare hashes, infused oils, and weed-infused spices, *Bong Appétit* (the show) redefines luxury in many respects. We realize that many readers, even those who live in states such as California and Colorado where recreational cannabis is legal, won't have access to these products. So we've translated many ideas from the series into something that works for the home cook. Do you have access to terpenes, cannabinoids, distillates, tinctures, and any strain of bud

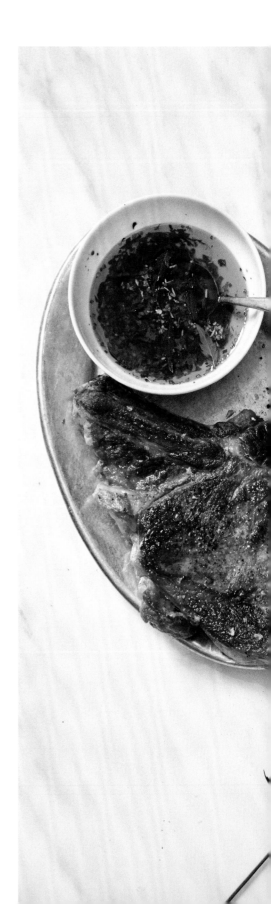

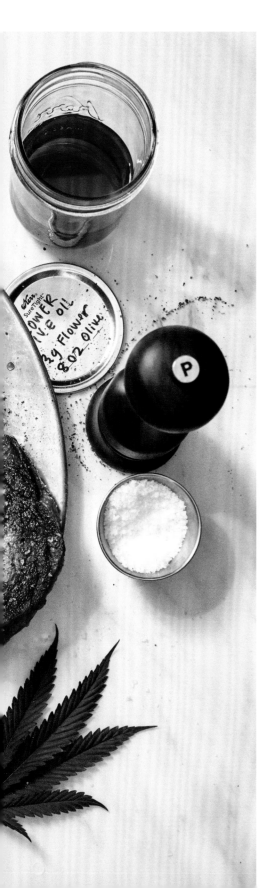

you desire and are looking for new techniques that will put them on your home table or turn them into professional-level edibles? These recipes will give you plenty to work with. Do you have to text someone shady as hell to get hooked up, so you basically have to work with whatever you can get? There are recipes here for you, too.

And we're making it easy to know just how high you'll get from a plate of fried chicken wings (see page 166) or a bowl of pappardelle Bolognese (see page 149). We lab tested all of our recipes to make sure you wouldn't have to worry about (a) wasting a bunch of weed making food that doesn't get you high or (b) making food that gets you so high you have to call in sick for work the next day. We've also asked *Bong Appétit* hosts Vanessa Lavorato and Ry Prichard to add notes and pro tips throughout the book so you get perspective from seasoned experts.

And sure, there's some crazy shit in here, like poaching a whole octopus in weed olive oil or force-infusing THC into alcohol with a whipped-cream charger. But we're also keeping it simple enough for the beginner cook to play along, with cannabis getting into most of the recipes via easy-to-make infusions of butter or oil. Still, if you're itching for a challenge, you'll find plenty of next-level options, from cannabis-leaf kimchi to infused pepperoni.

Some of what you may have seen on the show flies in the face of the conventional wisdom that prioritizes budget over flavor when cooking with weed. We freely admit that burning three ounces of high-quality pot in a smoker or dumping a handful of herb into a fryer was more about experimentation than getting high. You won't find recipes for that kind of thing here. That said, if you feel like balling out, we're not here to stop you. This book is all about giving you the tools and savvy you need to master the art of cooking with cannabis—no matter what that looks like for you.

If you live in a place without legal weed, please know we're sorry—and that you are not alone. And, yes, it's incredibly fucked up that there are millions of people in prison for enjoying the kind of recreational activity you're about to read an entire book on, and we're hoping that changes soon too. In any case, rest assured that the recipes in this book can be followed without including any cannabis at all. They're still excellent; they're just not quite as fun.

Equipment

Sadly, not everyone can live in cannabis-friendly Los Angeles with an elaborately outfitted pot pantry in their kitchen like on *Bong Appétit*. On the bright side, you don't need much more than your basic kitchen essentials—plus a good dispensary or a good dealer—to cook with weed. So in addition to the usual pots and pans, knives, spoons, and bowls, here is what you will need.

Canning jars: Vital for using the jar method for infusing. The size you need depends on what you are infusing, so keep an array of different sizes in your cupboard, as well as backup lids and bands. When used in boiling water, the lids and bands can degrade quickly and put your precious cannabis oils at risk of becoming waterlogged.

Cheesecloth: Essential for straining cannabis plant matter out of finished infusions.

Digital kitchen scale: Reliable measurements are especially important when dealing with cannabis flowers, kief, and extracts to ensure correct dosing. Look for a high-quality scale capable of precise measurements down to the milligram.

Instant-read thermometer: Cannabis infusions require attention to temperature throughout the process, making our instant-read thermometer the gift that keeps on getting us high.

Mesh strainers: Indispensable for creating infusions. Having mesh strainers on hand in a variety of sizes is a good idea as it will allow you to work at any scale.

Microplane grater: This fine-rasp grater is ideal for grating tiny bits of hash or flower over finished dishes. It is also especially helpful if you're working with compressed chunks of hash.

Rubber spatulas: For scraping every bit of THC-laced batter out of a bowl.

Once you have the basics on hand, you will want to think about some nice-to-have options.

Coffee grinder: If you're cooking with weed frequently, or need to grind up larger quantities of weed that would overload a simple herb grinder, a dedicated coffee grinder is very helpful.

Dab tools: If you anticipate doing a lot with cannabis extracts, you might want a set of dab tools—little spoons, pokers, and angled sharp-edged implements—plus a bottle of isopropyl alcohol for getting your tools clean. "Iso" can be bought at a pharmacy and has a number of household uses—grease remover, disinfectant, glass cleaner—precisely what you need to clean sticky dab tools as well as gunky glass pipes and dirty grinders. Buy tools sold as "wax carving sets," rather than branded cannabis-specific dab tools, to save some cash (but still make sure they are stainless steel or titanium).

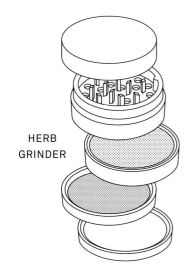

HERB GRINDER

Herb grinder: Cannabis flowers are generally ground before rolling a joint or loading a bowl, so a whole array of cannabis-specific devices known as herb grinders exist. Resembling a big hockey puck, these grinders are made of metal, wood, or plastic and have top and bottom halves, with an interior lined with spikes. The herb is placed inside the grinder and the top and bottom are turned back and forth between your hands until the herb is ground. The grinder is then opened and the contents are tapped out onto a rolling surface. You can use a herb grinder for cooking purposes, too, especially for small-scale applications. Grinders from Sweetleaf, Mendo Mulcher, and Santa Cruz Shredder work wonders. Go for a metal one, over plastic or wood, as the teeth are far stronger and the (hopefully) super-sticky herb you're loading into it is less likely to gum it up and break the teeth.

Parchment paper: Useful for storing sticky cannabis oils, parchment also has a variety of uses in a cannabis kitchen, from lining pans for baking cookies to pressing rosin.

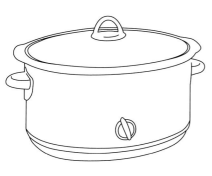

SLOW COOKER

Silicone baking mats: Sticky hash won't cling to silicone, so get a variety of sizes of silicone baking mats, traditionally used for lining sheet pans for baked goods. Now manufactured for the

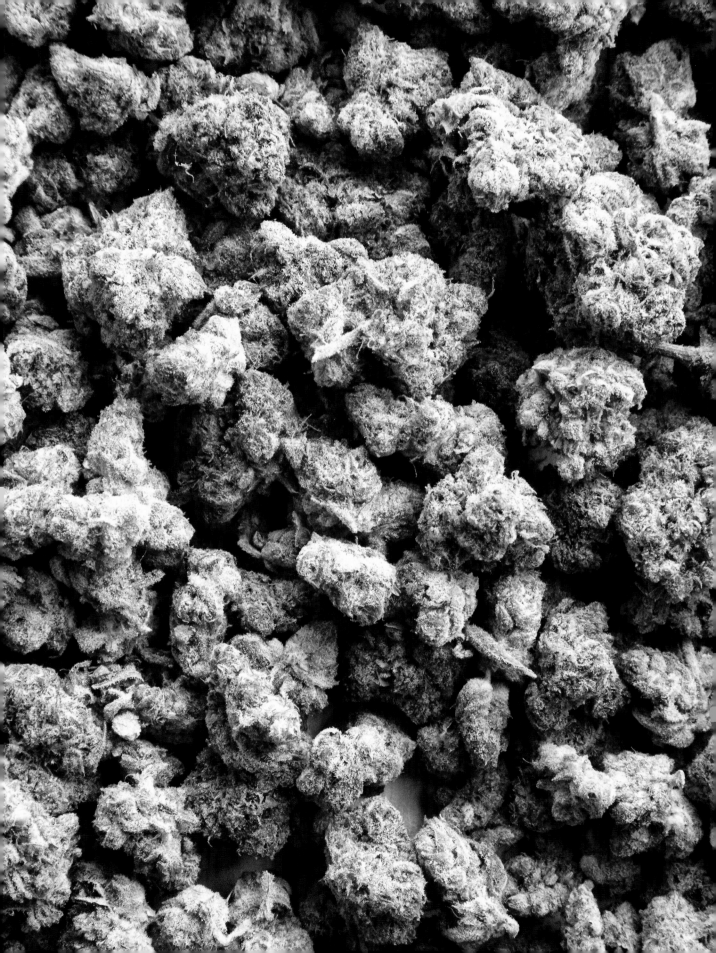

cannabis market by a variety of companies, these mats help keep surfaces free of difficult-to-clean oil stains but also make it easy to handle some of the more-tacky consistencies.

Slow cooker: Handy for simmering infusions for a long time at a low temperature.

Spice ball or tea strainer: A large, spherical spice ball or tea strainer is convenient for cannabis infusions, as you can add the weed to the strainer, immerse it in a big pot of oil or melted butter, and then easily remove it later.

If you're serious about cooking with weed, here's a bunch of transcendent equipment to acquire.

Automatic infusion machine: Set-it-and-forget-it infusion machines are the future, with several appliances on the market that remove the guesswork from infusing cannabis flowers or extracts into fats, glycerin, or alcohol. Some of the most advanced infusion machines can even strain out the cannabis material afterward, making the whole process a truly simple, low-mess affair. Two well-known brands are the MagicalButter machine, which has settings for creating infusions and tinctures with different kinds of fat, and the elegant LEVO machine, which infuses cannabis into oil or melted butter and then even strains it for you.

Decarboxylation machine: If you really want to live large, buy a dedicated decarboxylation machine. The NOVA decarboxylator is a brilliant new invention that activates THC precisely.

Grape press: This device is normally used to juice grapes, but you can also use it to juice the last little bit of cannabinoid content out of your infusion material.

Smoke gun and pellet smoker: You can add smoke to food by using a smoke gun or pellet smoker (though you need a lot of cannabis to make a pellet smoker work); both methods are more about adding flavor than actually getting weed into things. If a little smoky flavor and some tableside flash are all you want, you can pipe smoke under a cloche to dress up oysters on ice.

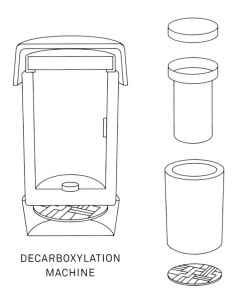

DECARBOXYLATION
MACHINE

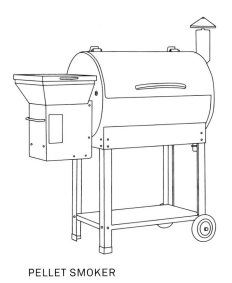

PELLET SMOKER

The Pot Pantry

The *Bong Appétit* pot pantry is huge, wildly expensive, and awe-inspiring. A walk-in weed closet tucked into the corner of the show's test kitchen, it houses more than thirty types of high-end cannabis strains, a dizzying array of hash and extracts, and tons of other infused and concentrated ingredients like oils, spices, terpenes, and distillates—all collected directly from California's finest producers. It's basically the equivalent to having a fully-stocked private dispensary on hand at all times, only with a wider selection and more cutting-edge options.

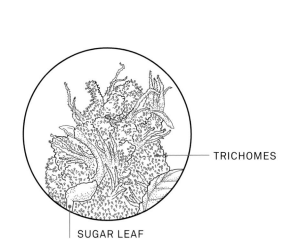

Obviously, you don't need all that to get started cooking with weed. But it doesn't hurt to know what's out there before diving in. Let's start with the most familiar forms of cannabis and then get weirder.

Flower

The form of dried cannabis that's typically ground and rolled into a joint or smoked in a pipe is known as "flower" since it is literally the flowers of the cannabis plant. The plant itself is unique because it produces both male and female flowers, with the former pollinating the latter. However, only female cannabis flowers produce significant amounts of the high-inducing cannabinoid THC found in the plant's resin, so growers typically separate females from males early in the cultivation process and allow them to mature to their full splendor without ever going to seed.

Depending on the variety and its growing conditions, flower—sometimes called "bud," "nugget," or just "nug"—can vary widely in potency from 10 to 30 percent THC content, with variation

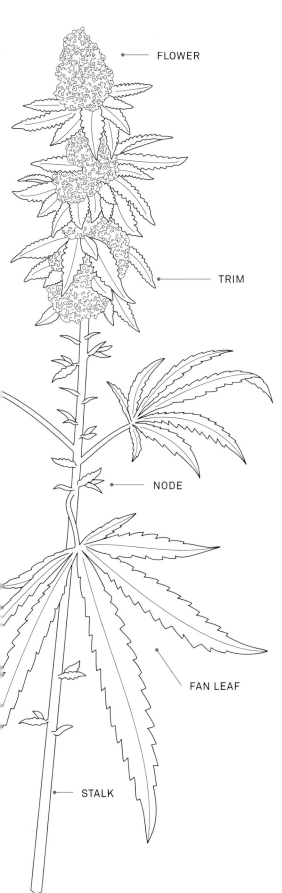

FLOWER

TRIM

NODE

FAN LEAF

STALK

found even within different parts of the same plant. The biggest bud on top of a plant is called the "cola," and it receives the most energy from light. That means it grows larger and generally has a higher quantity of the desirable psychoactive resin than do the smaller buds on the lower branches. Typically, the best buds are dried, cured, and reserved for smoking, while the smaller, less-potent "popcorn nugs" that appear toward the often-shaded bottom and center of the plant are relegated to culinary use or extraction. As cannabis costs fall with the increase in legal production, cooks will be able to source and utilize different and higher-quality cannabis ingredients. That includes flowers cultivated using specific methods (e.g., organic, vegan), the sourcing of specific varietals that offer special aromatic or flavor qualities, and also the utilization of high-flavor or high-potency cannabis extracts.

Why are cannabis extracts better culinary ingredients than flower? Well, all green parts of the cannabis plant contain chlorophyll, responsible for the "grassy" taste most people associate with weed food. Refining flowers into hash or extracts before use in food removes most, if not all, of this chlorophyll and makes for a tastier, more-refined final product.

Flower can be used in cooking when it is freshly harvested (especially for juicing), but is generally utilized after it has been dried and cured for smoking. Cannabis flower won't get you high on its own as it needs to be decarboxylated (exposed to heat) for the THCA present in the flower to be converted into THC, its psychoactive form. Once activated, the decarboxylated cannabis needs to be infused into fats, sugars, or alcohol, although technically it can be eaten on its own and still have an effect. (On the show, they frequently crisp broken flowers in fat and then use the cooked bud fragments to garnish other dishes.)

Trim

Also known as "sugar leaf," *trim* is the industry term for the small leaves, near the buds, that are trimmed away when flowers are manicured for sale after harvest. Traditionally used for making cost-effective edibles, trim contains significant amounts of THC

Comparison of Raw Cannabis Ingredients (Option 1)

Type of Cannabis Ingredient		THC Percentage by Weight	THC Content	Acidic THC Content
Flower: Forbidden Fruit strain (dried and cured)		9.05	3.2 mg/g	99.5 mg/g
Trim: Forbidden Fruit strain (dried and cured)		3.68	2.4 mg/g	39.2 mg/g
Kief: Forbidden Fruit strain		55	44.6 mg/g	584 mg/g

and other cannabinoids that would otherwise be wasted. Considered too harsh for smoking and too fibrous just to eat, these leaves can be used to make hash or infused directly into fats for cooking. High-quality trim can test up to 15 percent THC, with lower-quality samples measuring between 2 and 5 percent THC, making it a much-lower-potency product than flower.

Like flower, trim can be used fresh and raw or after being dried and cured. Also like flower, trim must be decarboxylated before its THC content is fully available. Trim delivers more chlorophyll because the plant matter has been snipped apart, often creating a grassier taste when infused, compared to flower.

Fan Leaves

The large, iconic cannabis leaves gather solar energy for plant growth, which means they contain copious amounts of chlorophyll and only trace amounts of THCA. Fan leaves are also fibrous and tough, so they can be hard to digest when fully grown. If you're looking to eat them raw in a pesto or salad, choose young, tender leaves from a plant in an early stage of growth; their flavor lands somewhere between kale and shiso, with slight variations in flavor based on the strain. Unfortunately, you can't buy a bag of baby pot leaves at Whole Foods yet, so you'll need to grow them yourself or source them directly from the farmer.

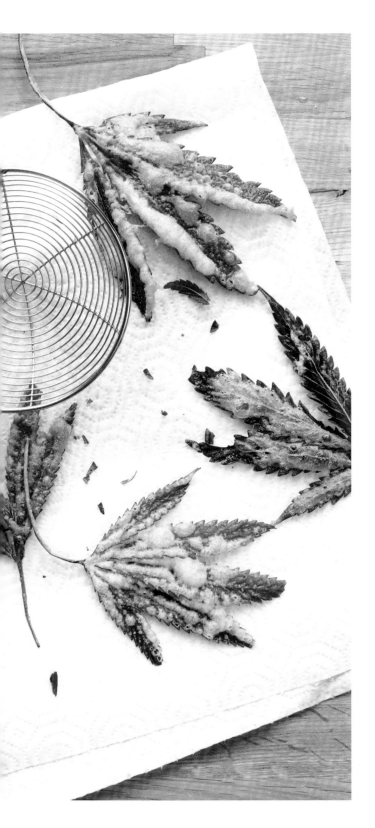

Although they're not recommended for edibles, fan leaves can be used for the cannabis leaf chips on page 220, the kimchi on page 234, and the candied leaves in "Vanessa Says" on page 211. Fan leaves can also be juiced for a rich source of acidic cannabinoids that won't get you high. The acidic precursor to THC is known as THCA, and it provides a variety of medicinal benefits, such as anti-inflammatory and anti-emetic properties, without psychoactive effects. The juice can be mixed into cocktails or frozen into ice pops. The most common use for fan leaves, however, is as a garnish or as part of a table decoration, as they really help your dinner party say, "This food has weed in it."

Leaves are highly perishable. Like any other fresh herb or cut flower, they begin to wither and dry out quickly if not kept in a properly humid environment. Wrap their stems in a damp paper towel, seal in a plastic bag, and then refrigerate to maintain freshness. You can also store the leaves or small shoots with stems in a glass of water in the fridge for a few days, like you do with cilantro or basil. Fan leaves are almost always used raw, and their THC content is so low as not to be worth trying to decarb for infusing.

Trichomes

While you won't see a container labeled "tri-chomes" in the *Bong Appétit* pantry, these tiny resin glands are scattered throughout the cannabis plant—particularly on its buds—where the majority of the plant's THC can be found. To the naked eye, these glands look like glittery crystals and they are responsible for the frosty appearance of top-shelf flower. When magnified, they look like sphere-topped stalks—crystal mushrooms from another planet. These resin-filled spheres are the most desirable part of the cannabis plant and are responsible for the vast majority of its effects, as well as its aroma and flavor, thanks to the rich essential oils packed into the heads. They are harvested and concentrated into hash and various types of extracts using a variety of techniques that involve solvents, such as CO_2 or butane, or ice water.

Considered a raw cannabis ingredient, trichomes that have been separated from the plant matter and collected en masse are referred to as "kief" (see following), which must be decarboxylated in order to develop its psychoactive THC content fully. The two traditional forms of hash, compressed bricks and balls, are made entirely of kief.

Kief

A sandlike, light brown powder, kief is one of the most traditional methods of concentrating cannabis, with origins stretching back thousands of years to the vast cannabis fields of India, Morocco, and Pakistan. Kief is simply a collection of trichomes that have been separated from the cannabis plant by "dry sifting"—shaking buds or trim so that the trichome glands fall through fine fabric or metal screens. You can collect kief at home, but it's easier to buy it at a dispensary, as accumulating enough kief to use for cooking would take quite a long time. Every time you grind a flower, kief is separated from the plant matter and either sticks to the inside of the grinder or appears as a fine powder on your rolling tray. Many herb grinder models include a "kief catcher," a chamber separated from the grinding compartment by an ultrafine screen. With each grind, a small amount of kief is deposited into this chamber for later use.

Kief is one of the most versatile ways to use cannabis as an ingredient, as it can be stirred into or sprinkled onto dishes just like most spices. But at fifteen dollars per gram, it is currently more expensive than saffron. Once cannabis is cultivated on a much larger scale, prices will likely fall and terpene-rich kief, which can carry the unique, vibrant flavors of various cannabis strains into every dish, will become much more widely available.

Although kief is considered a raw cannabis ingredient, it may have low amounts of psychoactive THC because it has often been dried and cured or otherwise handled enough to cause partial THCA conversion. To activate the THC in these dry-sifted trichomes fully, decarboxylation, or "toasting" the kief (see page 55), is required.

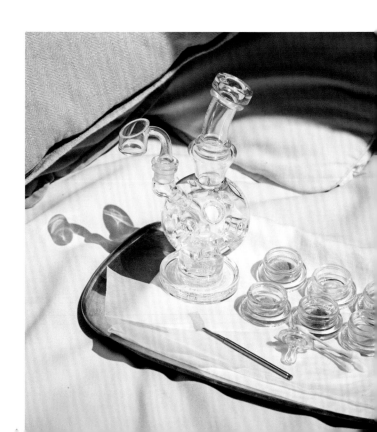

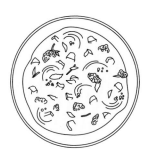

**1 - AGITATE CANNABIS
FLOWER WITH ICE WATER**

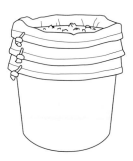

**2 - DRAIN THROUGH A SERIES
OF ICE-O-LATOR BAGS**

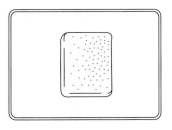

**3 — SPREAD OVER A BAKING
SHEET AND LET DRY**

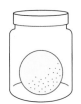

**4 — JAR AND CURE
BEFORE SERVING**

Water Hash

Hash is a catch-all term for concentrated and isolated trichomes prepared in a traditional fashion, either by dry sifting and then using a combination of heat and pressure, or by a water-based extraction method. Hash can appear as a granulated powder that looks like brown sugar, as pressed chunks of trichomes stuck together, or as a smooth, polished, potent temple ball, the age-old Nepalese form still created today by artisans such as Frenchy Cannoli.

While hash can be made using a variety of methods, the most common modern technique for physically separating trichomes from plant matter is known as water, or ice, hash. When cannabis flowers and/or trim are agitated together with ice water, the trichomes grow brittle and break off from the plant matter. Though water hash is commonly made using dried plant material, artisans have also started using fresh frozen plants, which many believe provide a much stronger aroma and flavor due to the higher concentrations of terpenes. Next, the loose trichomes are separated from the water by passing the water through a set of increasingly fine-mesh microscreen bags. The resulting mass is collected, dried, and cured, at which point it is ready for smoking or cooking. Some hash makers grate these chunks on a Microplane grater to increase surface area, speed drying, and prevent mold from forming in the interior. Water hash is known by several different names, including *ice wax*, *bubble hash*, and *full melt*.

Hash usually needs to be decarboxylated before cooking to fully activate all of its THC content. In its raw form, it does often contain a small percentage of THC, however, created during the

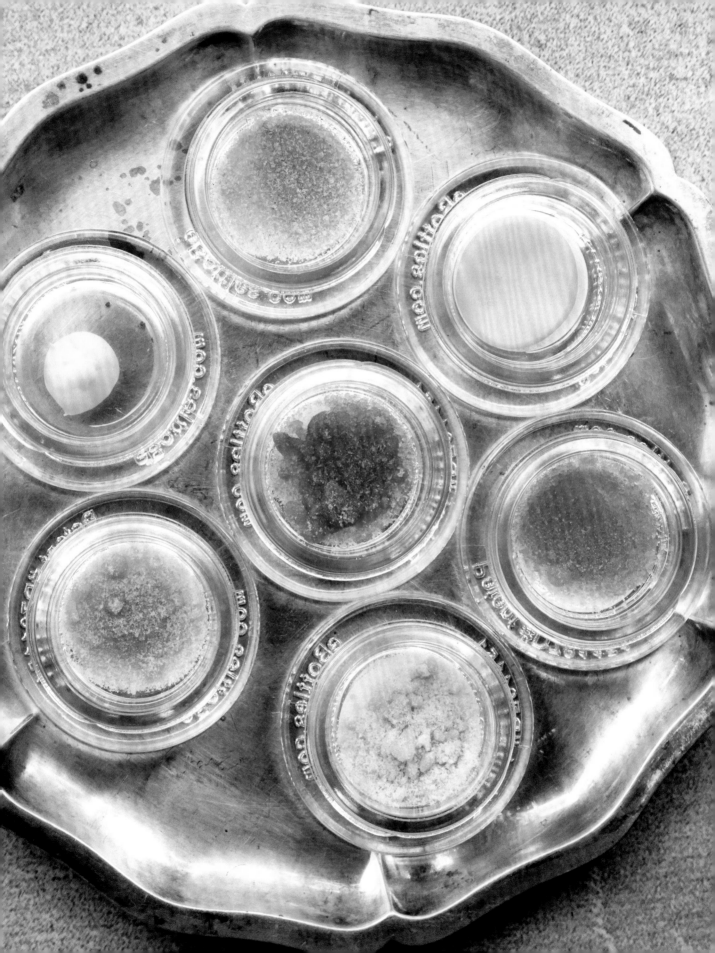

drying and curing process. You can use water hash in any recipe that calls for kief, but you'll need to grate it or crumble it into a fine powder to ensure even distribution. A Microplane grater is the best tool for working with hard chunks of hash, while other types crumble easily when chopped with a knife.

The best hash has amazing varietal-specific flavor that can greatly enhance the flavor of dishes. Medium- and lower-grade hash is still a more pure and concentrated form of cannabis compared to flower, and generally provides a cleaner, less obtrusive flavor free of the harsh, bitter, chlorophyll taste that can come from flower.

Concentrates and Extracts

Highly concentrated cannabis extracts are made by using either hydrocarbon solvents or CO2 to strip all the stuff that doesn't get you high from the stuff that does. What remains is a resinous extract of ultrapure cannabinoids, terpenoids, and flavonoids, which come in a bunch of different textures based on the post-extraction processes.

These extracts are primarily consumed via "dabbing," which means scooping up a small amount and then dropping it on a heated surface attached to a water pipe known as a "dab rig." Extracts can also be consumed in vaporizers, with the portable cartridge pen–style units being the most popular.

Cooking with extracts is a rare treat; it allows you to dose your food and control cannabis flavors incredibly precisely. Extracts are expensive

High-end water hashes from Rezn Extracts display a variety of colors and textures. Clockwise from top: Fine-grade Elmer's Glue, Cookies rosin, Candyland, a coarser grade of Elmer's Glue, Sour Grapes, Kosher Kush rosin, and Cookies.

(sometimes ranging from $60 to more than $100 per gram) and precious, so you probably won't be cooking with them all that often.

Following are the most common types of extracts on the market.

- **BHO**, short for *butane hash oil*, is made by using butane as a solvent to dissolve cannabinoids away from plant matter. Propane or other mixed-gas blends can also be used in the same way. This method of extraction is used in many industries, including for aloe, aspirin, and perfumes. BHO extracts generally contain between 65 and 80 percent THCA content.

- **Budder** or **Wax** is an opaque texture created through a post-extraction whipping process that creates an emulsion along with other aroma and flavor compounds such as terpenes. The texture gives the product its name; a softer, smoother, stickier consistency is generally referred to as "budder," while a drier, more crumbly consistency is known as "wax" or "crumble."

- **Distillates** are tasteless, odorless, up to 99 percent pure, and are often used for edible products in which no cannabis taste is desired. Distillate is extracted through a basic chemical evaporation process similar to the way alcohol is refined, with each step removing more impurities and undesired compounds. THC and CBDA distillate are the most common distillates found on the market.

- **Isolate** is any single molecule extraction, usually THCA or CBD. It generally comes in a crystalline form and is grown in a scientific glass vessel; just like those crystal kits you had as a kid. While incredibly useful for precise dosing of edibles, isolate is devoid of any other cannabinoids or terpenes, leading to a highly singular effect that many argue lacks the character (and sometimes medicinal qualities) of a multimolecule product.

- **Live resin** is a terpene-rich extract from freshly harvested plants that are quickly frozen, ideally using a cryogenic freezer. By capturing the plant at its aromatic peak, the extractor is able to create a concentrate with higher percentages of terpenes than a product made from dried plant material. Live resin is made using butane or propane, though there is also "live rosin" or "frosin," which is rosin made using fresh-frozen kief that has been sifted away from the plants. Live resin can take many forms, including budder, crystalline, sauce, shatter, and sugar, depending on how it is handled post-extraction. Live resin tends to have less THCA than concentrates made from dry material because it has more terpenes in the mix, so it generally tests between 60 and 75 percent THCA.

- **Rosin** is created from either flowers or hash, which are extruded into a concentrate using just pressure and heat. At-home hash-makers tend to utilize hair straighteners for small-batch production, though many companies have begun selling large-scale extractor units capable of tons of pressure and with customizable heat settings, allowing extractors to find the perfect press. Rosin can be made from dry or fresh-frozen material, though the latter is usually created from kief or water hash because fresh buds cannot

be pressed cleanly. While it has seemingly just come into vogue in the last couple of years, rosin is actually based on an ancient African extraction process involving conical baskets and heat from the sun. The texture of rosin can be clear like shatter but tends to become opaque quickly and ends up with a budder, wax, or sugary consistency. Like most extracts, it can take on almost any texture with varying amounts of heat and pressure. Rosin is usually between 55 and 75 percent THCA, though some extractors have figured out a way to separate out 99+ percent pure THCA using rosin-based processes.

- **Sauce** is a newer texture that has stolen the spotlight, thanks in large part to its gorgeous appearance. It's a mix of THCA crystals of varying size (often called "diamonds" when they reach a certain size and distinctness) floating in a "sauce" of extremely aromatic terpenes and flavonoids between 30 and 50 percent THCA. This sauce portion is often referred to as HTFSE, or high terpene full spectrum extract, while the crystal portion is often called HTFCE, or high terpene full cannabinoid extract.

- **Shatter** is a clear concentrate generally made using BHO processes, though rosin sometimes takes on this consistency as well. Shatter can be very brittle and break apart like glass (hence the name) or it can be more sticky like sap, depending on the terpenes present in the extract and also the ambient temperature. To make sappy shatter brittle and easier to handle, you can cool it by placing it between two cold surfaces. Shatter is usually between 60 and 80 percent THCA, depending on quality.

Comparison of Raw Cannabis Ingredients: Flower, Trim, and Kief

Type of Cannabis Ingredient	THC Percentage by Weight	THC Content	Acidic THC Content
Flower: Forbidden Fruit strain (dried and cured)	9.05	3.2 mg/g	99.5 mg/g
Trim: Forbidden Fruit strain (dried and cured)	3.68	2.4 mg/g	39.2 mg/g
Kief: Forbidden Fruit strain	55	44.6 mg/g	584 mg/g

Dabbing concentrate onto a hot surface or smoking flower by burning it instantly decarboxylates it before the resulting smoke is inhaled. Cannabis extracts and flower must both be decarboxylated for cooking in order to activate THC fully, and you can do this by toasting them in the oven (see page 55), heating in a saucepan, or with the "sous vide" method (see page 58) or jar method (used in chapter 1). The only exception to this rule is THC distillate, which is already activated and can simply be added to recipes or consumed directly.

Terpenes

Naturally occurring chemical components found in cannabis and many other plants, terpenes are what make weed smell (and taste) the way it does. They can be citrusy, skunky, piney, or just straight-up dank. Terpenes from cannabis strains can be isolated and bottled, capturing the plant's essence for adding to drinks or dishes to imbue them with a distinct cannabis flavor but no high.

Used in cooking just like essential oils derived from plants such as mint or basil, these compounds deliver sensorial delights without any of the usual psychoactive effects of cannabis. It's worth mentioning with terpenes that a little goes a long way—one drop of terpenes can, at times, be enough to flavor an entire dish, depending on the strain's flavor profile and pungence. Terpenes can be purchased online, but cannabis-derived terpenes are expensive and exist in a somewhat gray legal area. You can easily find terpenes derived from other sources (such as pine trees or lemons), but these are not necessarily recommended for smoking or even adding to food because they are primarily created for aromatic applications such as aromatherapy atomizers. Make sure to read the labels for any terpenes to determine the types of use for which the specific product was created.

Terpenes (which are explored in-depth starting on page 43) provide the "flavor profile" of a cannabis strain, allowing for both the art and science of pairing weed strains (like wines) with food and for incorporating a specific strain into a recipe (like the Double-Lemon Roast Chicken on page 165 made with Lemon Skunk strain).

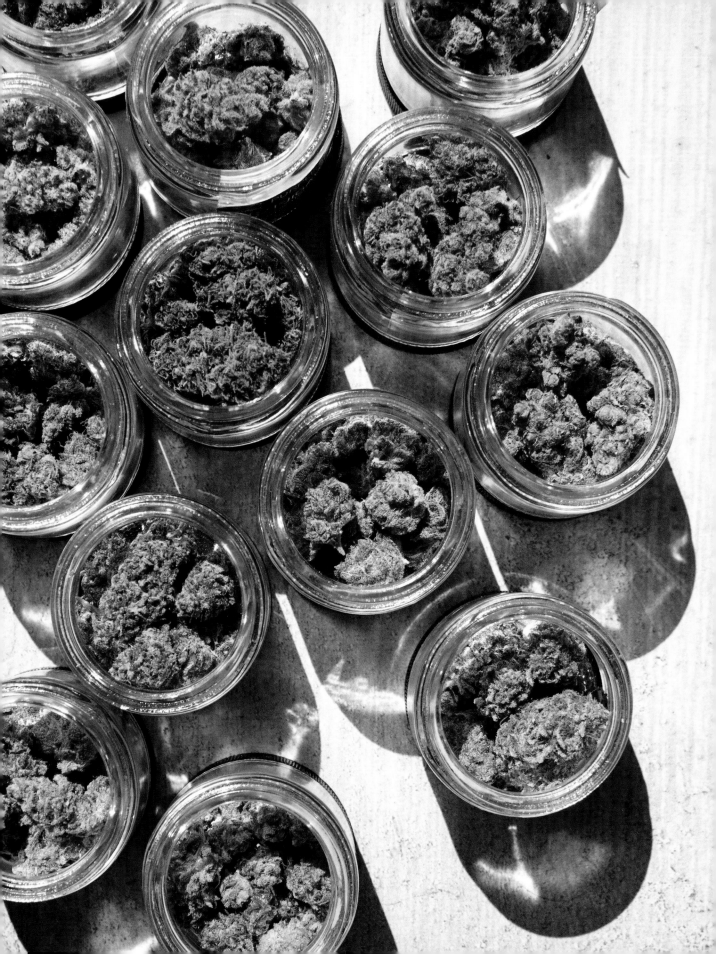

How to Go Weed Shopping

Wandering into a dispensary can be a little intimidating, even for the practiced pothead. Jars full of fuzzy, sparkling flowers in various shades of green; small containers of translucent amber extracts; and prepackaged edibles of every possible variety crowd the shelves, making it tough to determine exactly what you need—especially if you're new to cooking with cannabis. Based on your budget, you'll be looking to buy kief, hash, extracts, infused oils or butters, flowers, or trim for cannabis cooking projects. So whether it's the first time you've been to the pot store or it's your 420th visit, here's how to pick the perfect pot.

Bud Basics: Sativa vs. Indica

The distinctions between the two basic subspecies of cannabis—sativa and indica—have perhaps been overstated, especially since most of what's on the market is actually a hybrid of the two. It's basically a cliché that sativa strains are stimulating and cerebral, better for creative work or gaming, while an indica delivers a more relaxing or sedating body high.

Over the years, growers have crossed the two types extensively, looking for best-of-both-worlds progeny. Such hybrid strains have come to dominate the market so thoroughly that when a varietal is described as either sativa or indica, it's most likely an indicator of which genetics are dominant in the cross.

That said, some people respond much differently to sativa-dominant strains than to indica-dominant strains. And if that's

These award-winning cannabis flowers from Purple Frost Genetics have subtle differences from bud to bud.

you, definitely source the one that matches the mood you'd like to set. Heading out for a hike through the wilderness? Sativa. Wanting to unwind after a long day at work? Indica. Try to source varieties as close to 100 percent of one or the other to emphasize the desired effect.

At the time of writing, there is no legal or regulatory mechanism that requires producers to prove if a strain is sativa or indica; the genetics of most marijuana strains are murky at best. That means your best bet is to chat with the employees at your dispensary to figure out what is what.

How to Know What You'll Like

How do you know which weed is the one for you? You'll smell it! The type of cannabis that smells best to you is almost always the one with a high that you'll enjoy.

Increasingly, research points to the presence and combination of different terpenes as significantly influencing the effects of various strains. That means the future of cannabis classification is going to be much more complex and multifaceted than our current sativa/indica dichotomy. The distinction between the two is more relevant to cultivators and breeders, while consumers should begin to focus on the varying terpene profiles and "strain fingerprints" that truly determine how the variety makes them feel a certain kind of stoned.

For instance, it seems like strains with a significant amount of limonene (see page 50) tend to confer a high that's uplifting and creative—an effect traditionally attributed to the sativa subspecies.

How Legitimate Are Strain Names?

Literally tens of thousands of named cannabis strains exist, and 90 percent of the excitement around specific strains is little more than marketing hype. Sorry to burst anyone's bubble, but dispensary staff will randomly change the name of a strain to something that sounds better if pounds aren't moving out the door.

Say you have a friend in Santa Cruz who grows weed, and she gives you an amazing jar of Black Cherry Pie that smoked awesomely, smelled terrific, and gave you a great high. Seeking to replicate the experience while traveling, you go to a dispensary in Denver and buy some Black Cherry Pie, only to be disappointed when it doesn't give you the same type of high.

That scenario happens all of the time, and it's because the experience of a specific strain isn't just about the genetics. It's also about the *terroir* (the land and environmental factors affecting a crop) and the skill of the cultivator. The Black Cherry Pie you liked so much should really be called "Sarah's Santa Cruz Black Cherry Pie, Plant #207, Harvested on October 27," and it might have resonated with you because the terpene profile was expertly preserved during the curing process, an organic fertilizer regimen allowed the plant to express its best flavors fully, and the production of resin glands (trichomes) was maximized under the bright California sun during an exceptional Santa Cruz season. Much like wine, cannabis will smell, taste, and produce different effects depending upon how it is grown and handled throughout its life cycle. A grower can cultivate "the perfect plant" only to have it stored and cured improperly by someone down the line, which can totally destroy the flavor and smoking experience. Each step of the process is as important as the one that came before it.

Cannabis strains are created by growers and breeders, much like tomato or rose varieties in traditional horticulture. When done properly, seed breeding involves selecting for the hardiest plants most capable of thriving in a specific environment, or for plants that have a unique flavor profile, and the process of honing in on the best specimens is refined over many years. To have the most value as a consistent identifier, you must source strains directly from the breeder. Get your genetics from a reputable seed bank, such as Barney's Farm, Sensi Seeds, Crockett Family Farms, or DNA Genetics, and you're much more likely to find the consistent cannabis you're looking for.

With this understanding, when you're seeking to replicate a previously enjoyed high, either source from the same producer or seek out the same genetics grown in the same region in the original style. Or just trust your nose and smoke or eat the weed that smells the best to you.

Clone-Only vs. Seed Varieties

Another key piece of understanding why a certain cannabis strain makes you feel a certain way is knowing the difference between clone-only and from-seed plants. For example, the strain Golden Goat is a specific individual plant, chosen by the breeder from a handful of seeds and preserved via cloning, or asexual propagation, since the late 2000s. In exactly the same way cuttings are taken from tomato plants,

growers take cuttings from cannabis "mother plants" in order to create exact genetic replicas of their favorite varieties. This allows for repeatable results across a large number of plants, making it easier to dial in the way strains are grown, as well as produce a lot of one specific product. Most strains on dispensary shelves are actually just individual plants chosen by their grower and kept over time.

In contrast, varieties such as Super Lemon Haze, White Widow, and Deadhead OG have been released by seed companies. This means there are now literally thousands of different plants called "Super Lemon Haze" that resulted from the same parents, but all of which still have the potential to express different traits. While good breeders are able to produce seeds that provide a fairly repeatable experience, genetically there is still a huge variety of possibilities contained within each individual seed, making it difficult for a customer to know what they are getting every time. If you're not familiar with a strain, ask the dispensary for its lineage and whether it is clone-only or from seed; you will then have a better idea of how repeatable your experience will be with that particular variety.

How to Know If the Weed Is Good

If you are unable to officially hammer down the strain that you're smoking, the least you can do is make sure that whatever it is, it's good-quality. Always ask if you can open jars and sniff the merchandise because scent is usually the best indication of quality cannabis. Pass on any offering that smells musty or of harsh chemicals. These indicators can mean that a strain wasn't flushed properly before harvest, or that it was rushed to market and may have gotten moldy along the way because it wasn't properly dried and cured.

But if your test meets with a strong, pleasant aroma, then it's reasonable to assume the pot was grown and processed correctly. What you're smelling are the terpenes—THC doesn't have much of a smell on its own—and they are the best way to determine quality flowers.

Next, use a magnifying glass or microscope—which a dispensary or real overachiever of a dealer should have handy—to look at the quality and preservation of the trichomes and confirm the absence of mold, which looks like fuzzy white or gray patches. Using your naked eye, look at the bud for signs of discoloration as well as gouges from overzealous trimmers. While the presence of some leaf is okay, modern cannabis is trimmed thoroughly for a reason; the presence of leaf matter makes for a harsher smoke, so look for well-trimmed buds that are free of "crow's feet" leaves curling around the sides. Finally, the buds should ideally be sticky and firm to the touch, yielding to a slight squeeze. They should not be so dry that they break apart under slight pressure, although you can still consume bud in that condition. Storing cannabis properly in dry environments is especially important, as a place like Colorado with low relative humidity can turn a properly squishy bud into a dust pile waiting to happen in a matter of hours.

The dispensary staff is usually not going to let you touch or handle buds, so you can ask the budtender to squeeze it with their gloved hands for you.

Looking for trim? All the same tips apply as far as inspecting for mold and trusting your nose. Some dispensaries sell trim, and others don't, so call ahead to make sure. The best source for trim is from a friendly grower or your own plants. While it generally is less pungent-smelling than buds, trim should still have a distinct aroma and should never smell like hay or vegetation. Look for the presence of visible trichomes, and always ask if the trim is "hand trim" as opposed to "machine trim," as a hand-trimmed product is handled more carefully and usually has far-higher cannabinoid content.

When sourcing kief, ask if you can smell it and inspect for mold. Kief should be a light sandy color; a green tint indicates a sub-par extraction process that introduced too much plant matter. When evaluating other concentrates, ask the staff who crafted the concentrate, as well as what solvent was used. Concentrates (other than whole-plant ethanol-extracted oil intended for oral ingestion, often called RSO, or Rick Simpson Oil) should never be black or green. Extracts are generally of acceptable quality when they are white, golden, orange, or amber, and they should also smell distinctly like the strain(s) from which they were extracted. Many dispensaries will be able to provide you with lab test results for their products that show the cannabinoid content (THCA, THC, CBD, CBN usually) as well as residual solvents for concentrates (expressed in parts per million), and even the individual terpenes present in the sample. Lab testing is not perfect and should not be the sole determining factor for quality but, along with these other tools, can help to inform your cannabis buying decisions.

WHAT TO ASK AT THE DISPENSARY

When you visit your dispensary, ask the following questions to ensure that you leave with exactly the product you want.

— What's fresh today?

You want a recent batch of cannabis, not something that's been sitting on the shelf for too long.

— Is there anything that smells like oranges or lemons?

If you usually like citrusy cannabis, start there. If you tend toward floral or sweet-smelling strains, ask for strains that give off those aromas.

— What's good for an active day? What's good for sleep?

Asking if a strain supports specific effects will help you find the product you most enjoy.

— What do you have for under fifty dollars per eighth?

Being specific about your price point can greatly speed up a consultation. Dispensary staff don't want to offer you options that you can't afford.

— Is this sun grown or indoor? Was it fed with traditional nutrients, or was it grown organically?

If you're looking for eco-friendly cannabis, make sure it was grown outdoors or in a greenhouse, which runs on much less energy than a warehouse full of high-intensity discharge lamps. Plus, cannabis nurtured in a living soil and fed compost can be much more flavorful. As you consume cannabis grown using different nutrients and in diverse growing mediums (soil, coco coir, mineral wool, pure hydroponic, aeroponic, etc.), you'll become more familiar with what you like and don't.

— Is this lab tested? Can I see a terpene profile?

Most dispensaries must test their cannabis for THC potency and to confirm products are free of pesticide residue. Some places also test for terpene profiles, but not all. So, for example, so if you're looking for a strain high in limonene, you might have to rely on your nose.

Get It Farm Fresh

There's an expanding organic-pot movement afoot, with master cannabis growers tailoring their cultivation methods to specific weed strains to coax the best aromas and flavors out of their bud. Just like farmers' market produce, pot from a good grower makes a world of difference.

Complicating the issue is the fact that the United States Department of Agriculture (USDA) determines what can be called "organic" via on-site inspection, and since cannabis is still illegal in the eyes of the federal government, it cannot be legally inspected, labeled, or sold as USDA organic.

Third-party certification services, including Clean Green, Certified Kind, and the Cannabis Certification Council, have sprung up to identify eco-friendly cannabis growers and distinguish their products from competitors, so be sure to ask your dispensary if it carries any cannabis that has been verified as environmentally sound.

Indoor vs. Outdoor

It's a common misconception that cannabis grown indoors is automatically superior to cannabis grown outdoors; songs about "indo" or "hydro" notwithstanding. The skill of the farmer and the quality of the plant's genetics is the main determining factor in whether or not cannabis is good, not just where it was grown.

The most photogenic and aromatic buds tend to come from indoor farms powered by high-intensity artificial lights (much like those hothouse tomatoes imported from Holland), which means they typically fetch premium prices at market. But there's also an increasing movement to support small, eco-friendly cannabis farmers raising "sun grown," or outdoor, weed. Many connoisseurs believe that the sun's rays cause the plants to produce different compounds and greatly increase their vigor, leading to a product that can have a higher medicinal and flavor potential when cultivated properly.

Much like the farm-to-table movement in food, going small and organic when buying weed allows you to incorporate top-quality herb into your cooking while supporting artisanal growers following best practices. With more brands available than ever before, do a little research into who grew your weed and where. The best weed is grown in small batches by people who care about it and who have honed their methods over years of experience. Much like craft brews, bean-to-bar chocolate, and fine wine, there are no shortcuts when it comes to growing, harvesting, drying, and curing primo weed.

Weed Storage

Once you get your cannabis home from the dispensary, you need to keep it as fresh as possible. Cannabis flowers, hash, and extracts all benefit from being stored in a cool, dry, dark place. Some connoisseurs store their extracts in a wine fridge, which helps preserve flavors and aromas that evaporate over time or when exposed to light and heat.

Choose an airtight, opaque glass jar for long-term storage of cannabis flowers and try to use your flowers within three months. Old cannabis will turn golden yellow, and its aroma loses nuance, becoming much like hay or old grass clippings.

Extracts also begin to degrade as they age depending on how they are stored, and many types of concentrate become more volatile. Both temperature and humidity can cause changes in consistency over time. High terpene extracts such as live resin and fresh frozen rosin are highly perishable because terpenes evaporate easily, so it's usually best to enjoy these products as quickly as possible.

The exception to the short-term storage rule is artisanally produced hashes and temple balls made in the traditional fashion, which can benefit from a long cure that develops flavor. Kief and most types of water hash should ideally be used within three months.

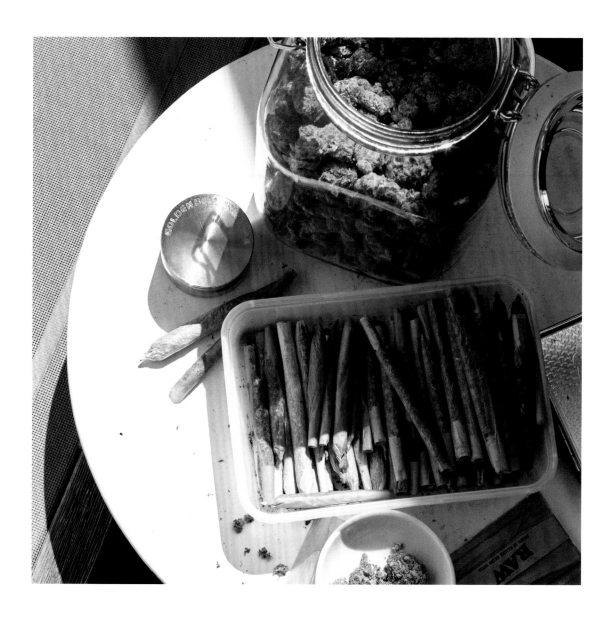

In the Cannabis Lab

In making and testing infusions for this book, we consulted with Dr. Jeff Raber from The Werc Shop, a prestigious cannabis lab in Southern California. The lab tests products using an analytical chemistry method known as high-performance liquid chromatography (HPLC), which can separate, identify, and quantify each component in a mixture. Without the benefit of the equipment that makes this technique possible, professional edibles manufacturers would be unable to determine THC content precisely.

So how can home cooks get the most bang for their buck out of weed? Dr. Raber says it helps to be methodical and pay attention to details every step of the way. "Standardization at home is exceptionally challenging," he explains. "There are a lot of variables on which you have no insight and no way to double-check."

For starters, are you working with any reliable test values whatsoever? Even if your cannabis is sold as having 25 percent THC, in reality that value might be much lower. "Is that test value representative of the 5 grams that you bought? Maybe; maybe not," Raber says.

Why is this? Well, the inherent nature of plant material is not homogeneous. Cannabis flowers have many little nooks and crannies where THC can hide, and there's variation in potency from the top of the plant, which gets a lot of light to maximize resin production, and the bottom of the plant, where flowers are less potent. All of this means that different parts of the same cannabis plant can vary from 15 to 25 percent THC.

Sparkling trichomes containing THC and other cannabinoids cover this batch of Platinum Girl Scout Cookies grown by Kyle Kushman.

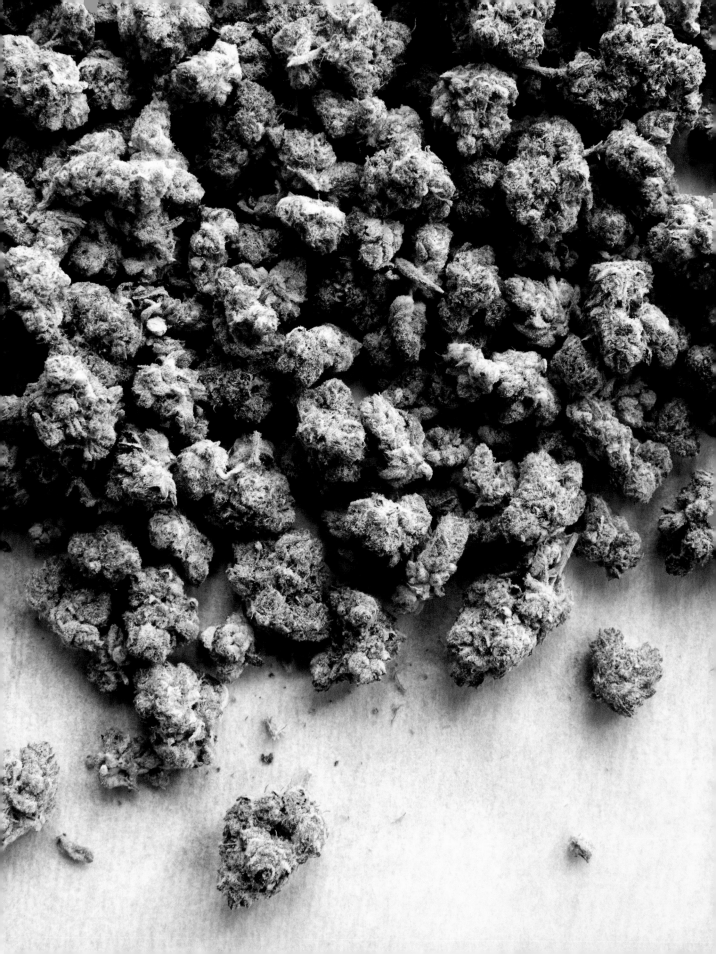

Concentrates are much more homogeneous due to the absence of plant matter, making them better suited to cooking consistent batches of edibles and estimating potency at home. Concentrates are also nice because you can use very small amounts thanks to their high potency levels, making it easier to hide the cannabis flavor if so desired. Also, despite their higher per-gram price, concentrates are generally almost the same value proposition as using flowers for cooking because you can use so little at a time.

As far as infusion methods, Raber says that "the mason-jar method is pretty efficient as far as we've seen. It depends on the heat and how long you do it, but I haven't been able to do a lot of tests on the spent plant material." Doing what's known as a "mass balance test" to measure the THC left behind is the only way to know if all of the cannabinoids were captured and how efficient the infusion was.

Cannabinoids

When we get lab test results, what we're looking for are the levels of different cannabinoids found in flowers, trim, kief, hash, and other ingredients used in a cannabis kitchen. The cannabis plant owes both its medicinal benefits and its pleasant high to a set of compounds called *cannabinoids* that are virtually unique to the species. Blending THC and CBD to desired effect is already established practice among cannabis-adept chefs, and every day our understanding of weed's remaining eighty-plus cannabinoids grows through experimentation.

Some cannabinoids, like THC, THCA, and CBD, can be found in isolated, purified forms, including crystalline and distillate extracts. When reading test results, other cannabinoids will be listed, and it's helpful to know their effects and properties when you're evaluating specific products. High amounts of CBDA and THCV are found in certain cannabis strains, with varying ratios present in all cannabis products derived from whole plants. Following are the most commonly known and studied cannabinoids, which can help boost your understanding of the scientific complexities of whole-plant medicine.

CBD Lesser known but gaining quickly in popularity, CBD is shorthand for cannabidiol. A non-euphoric component of cannabis, CBD has anti-inflammatory benefits and aids in muscle relaxation and lowering anxiety. CBD also tempers the anxiety that can sometimes result from THC, preventing it from becoming too overwhelming. High levels of CBD can be found in certain strains, such as Harlequin, ACDC, and Sour Tsunami, and its presence would also be in the extracts or infusions made from these strains.

CBDA The acidic form of CBD is present in freshly harvested high-CBD cannabis strains and can be made available through juicing or extraction. Like THCA and its activated form, THC, CBDA is converted to CBD via decarboxylation (heat and time) when infused or smoked.

CBG Cannabigerol (CBG) is a minor cannabinoid, but it seems to have a big impact on fighting tumor growth. It's also particularly effective at killing bacteria and reducing inflammation.

CBN Cannabinol (CBN) is a degraded form of THC and THCA that results from oxidation or UV light exposure. Heating your infusions for too long or at too high a temperature will cause the THC to convert into CBN, which is a known sedative. So if you're looking for a natural sleep aid, CBN is wonderful. Otherwise, it's usually a sign that you need to fine-tune your infusion process.

THC Short for Delta-9-tetrahydrocannabinol, this magic molecule is what started the love affair between humanity and weed. Responsible for the euphoria, giggles, and good times we all associate with being high, THC is the main psychoactive component in cannabis flowers, trim, kief, hash, and all types of products made with these ingredients.

THCA This is the inactive, acidic form of THC found in living plants, as well as cured buds and trim. While some hash and concentrates have small amounts of THC present, they are also primarily THCA, which becomes THC when smoked or decarboxylated for infusion. THCA possesses many of the same healing qualities as THC, but because it has not yet been "decarb'ed" (that is, decarboxylated), it is not psychoactive. Look for THCA in certain tinctures or capsule products formulated to possess healing effects without the psychedelic high of activated THC.

THCV A rarely occurring cannabinoid with an interesting effect, tetrahydrocannabivarin (THCV) may have appetite suppression properties, leading to conjecture that a strain of "skinny weed" could be created to actively encourage weight loss. Only a small percentage of strains have any THCV presence, but there may be many more that are just waiting to be discovered.

Dosing

First off, it's basically impossible to eat so much THC that you die. Colorado's recommended dose (which most other legal states have followed) for edibles is 10 milligrams of active THC per serving. It's estimated that a 175-pound man would need to eat 53 grams of pure THC in one sitting to reach a fatal dose. That's an occurrence so unheard-of as to be theoretical; as long as you aren't shooting tons of pure THC right into your bloodstream, you'll survive.

Although THC is much safer than alcohol, caffeine, and nicotine, it can definitely make your heart race, inducing anxiety and panic attacks if you eat too much, so go slowly and learn your limits. If you accidentally go overboard, it could take a while—and maybe a few freak-outs—before the fog begins to lift.

In states where pot is legal, store-bought edibles are routinely lab tested for potency and are accurately labeled with suggested serving sizes. Knowing the cannabinoid content has been a huge game changer for all of the people who swore off edibles forever after a bad experience. Even if you don't have access to a fancy weed lab, there are a few steps you can take to make sure your at-home dosing is manageable.

When making your own infusions, follow the instructions in this book carefully and be sure to double-check your math. And always round up when estimating THC content, assuming there is more pot in a recipe than you might think. Why? The difference between a very pleasant edibles experience and a very unpleasant one can hinge on consuming just 10 milligrams more THC than planned for, so why not err on the side of caution? You can always eat more; you can never eat less.

Vanessa Says: If you've never cooked with cannabis before, just keep in mind that a little can go a long way. It's easy to throw a bunch of flowers into butter and make a potent edible. Patience and restraint only means you get to eat more edibles until you find the right dose for you. My first time in the kitchen, I chose the other path. It was a 420 I'll never remember.

If you're in a legal state, you can skip a couple of steps here and just buy premade infusions. Weed-infused butters, oils, honeys, and chocolates are all widely available at finer pot shops and can easily be incorporated into a wide variety of recipes. Basically, it all comes down to how high you want to get. If you're looking for a gentle 10-milligram dose of THC, find a cannabis chocolate bar with segments dosed appropriately and then melt a piece into your hot cocoa. The same is true for honey: if 1 tablespoon delivers 10 milligrams, drizzle that amount into your tea.

From Microdosing to Greening Out

Finding your minimum effective dose is important, whether you're an experienced edibles consumer or a new user. Discovering the smallest possible amount of THC that causes you to feel effects is possible through trial and error, and knowing your dose will help you avoid having an unpleasant experience. Everyone's body chemistry varies greatly when it comes to the effects of cannabis consumption, and the right dose for you could range anywhere between 5 and 500 milligrams.

Your metabolism, fitness level, diet, and other factors come into play in how your body processes and tolerates edibles. For example, athletic people notice effects from smaller amounts of THC because their bodies operate at maximum efficiency. Cannabis works its way through your digestive system before ending up in the liver, where THC is converted into 11-hydroxy-THC, an even more potent chemical. This in-body chemical conversion doesn't take place when you smoke weed, and it is the reason why edibles are so much more potent and long-lasting than smoking. (When you smoke, the THC is instantly combusted, inhaled through your lungs, and then enters your bloodstream, bypassing your liver.)

A new user of cannabis should begin with no more than 10 milligrams of THC and then wait two hours before taking any more. If you barely feel 10 milligrams, that's fine. Either after two hours or the next time, you can work your way up to 15 or 20 milligrams. Just increase your dose slowly until you find your minimum effective dose.

If you usually buy edibles, you've probably noticed more and more products are intended for microdoses, starting between 2.5 and 5 milligrams of THC, which makes it easier to calibrate the right dose for you. And while you'll see some hella potent products containing up to 1,000 milligrams of THC on dispensary shelves, they're not single-serving doses. They're just cost-effective for people who can pace themselves (and if you're not one of them, you're best off steering clear).

We've designed the recipes in this book to yield individual portions that are satisfying without exceeding your dosage limit. Most of the yields have been adjusted to deliver 5 to 10 milligrams of THC, with explanations on how you can add more if desired. A few of the desserts are dosed slightly higher. That's because if you're going to be indulgent, it might as well be with sweets.

HOW TO EAT WEED FOOD: A BEGINNER'S PRIMER

1. **Start low.** We cannot emphasize this strongly enough. Start at 5 to 10 milligrams and go up slowly until you find your minimum effective dose.

2. **Go slowly.** The classic rookie mistake is eating a dose, eating another a half hour later because you don't feel anything, and then getting too high. Wait at least two hours before going back for seconds.

3. **No booze for beginners.** Yes, we have a cocktails chapter, but that's some expert-level stuff. Eating cannabis and being drunk at the same time is usually awful, unless you happen to love the spins. If you're going to do both, keep it low-key. Eat a tiny bit of THC and stick to just one glass of wine or beer until you know how the combination will make you feel.

4. **Balance THC with CBD.** CBD (see page 34) takes the edge off a THC high, while providing its own sedative and anti-anxiety effects. So ingesting an edible with a 1:1 ratio of THC to CBD will provide a much more chill experience than will THC alone.

5. **Eat real food too.** Eating a light snack immediately before or after an edible will help slow the onset of the effects of THC, as it will take longer to digest and absorb into your body. Conversely, eating weed on an empty stomach will intensify its effects.

6. **Label your THC treats.** Pot food is great. Accidentally eating pot food is the worst. Also, make sure your stash is kept safely away from children and pets.

What to Do If You Eat Too Much THC

Cannabis is a mild psychedelic, and if you've never tripped before, it can be unnerving. If you find yourself too damn high, here are a few proven strategies and anecdotal antidotes for making things right.

Black Peppercorns Chewing on one or two peppercorns (or even just inhaling the scent of freshly ground black pepper) can help assuage the paranoia brought on by too much THC. Beta-caryophyllene, a terpene found in pepper, actually binds to the cannabinoid receptors in your brain and produces a calming effect.

CBD Nonpsychoactive CBD (see page 34) acts to temper the high of THC by working on the same cannabinoid receptors in the brain and throughout the body. High-CBD vapes, tinctures, and edibles are available and will help you turn the corner if a high grows unmanageable.

Chill Don't stress. Nothing physically dangerous is happening. Find a quiet, dimly lit space and chill. Set an alarm if you need to wake up anytime in the next sixteen hours. Know that even if you get too baked, you will be able to sleep it off and wake up feeling a little groggy but okay.

Eat Food Eating something fatty, like a burger or fries, will help slow down the digestion of THC in your system and dilute the effects somewhat.

Stay Hydrated Drinking plenty of water helps flush the system, and fruit juice or a sugary beverage will raise your blood sugar so you feel more normal.

Vanessa Says: My advice is to make yourself comfortable, have all of your favorite munchies around, put on a funny movie, and relax. It'll pass. Of course, if you have a medical condition and are concerned, go to a doctor. But as far as I know, nobody has died from cannabis.

Things to Know About Dosing Cannabis Edibles at Home

For a great many science-based reasons, precisely dosing weed food cooked at home is incredibly difficult. Throughout this book, you'll see the potency of dishes estimated according to the lab results of our infused fats and other active ingredients. That means to replicate the dose level of a recipe at home, you'll need starting material of the same THC potency we used and to follow our directions for decarboxylation and infusion exactly.

Accounting for potential variables like THC potency is also why we made these recipes relatively low dose, so even if the THC dose has a 15 percent variation, it's still made for lightweights.

Why is it so hard to calculate THC doses in homemade edibles? Efficiency of decarboxylation and infusion methods are two reasons, and then you have to factor in that most foods aren't homogenous (especially if they are served "family style") and one part might end up more potent than another. Remember, raw cannabis contains THCA, the acidic version that must be heated to convert into psychoactive THC, so if you can't ensure all the THCA is converted to THC through the decarboxylation and infusion processes, that makes estimating dosage tricky. Theoretically, you should be able to say, "Well,

my cannabis tested at X percent THC, so if I put Y grams into Z pounds of butter, I'll get the perfect amount per 1 tablespoon."

That's a rough way to estimate dosage because it assumes that the maximum amount of THC available was extracted from the cannabis and that all of it got into the butter and was activated with 100 percent efficiency. It's a calculation that works only to determine the ceiling—in other words, it is the absolute most THC you can possibly get. In reality, you're reducing potency at every step of the process, as cannabinoids are lost or destroyed.

Calculating Potency of Homemade Infusions

According to our cannabis lab, the THCA present in cannabis converts to THC at a rate of 0.88 percent. Then, we have to consider the efficiency of our infusion method, which can vary from 40 to 60 percent when you're infusing cannabis flower into butter or oil. Infusions are inefficient because some THC gets vaporized in the process and some is lost in the straining, remaining in the plant material. Also, different types of fat absorb cannabis at different rates, so an oil rich in saturated fats (such as coconut oil) tends to be the most effective for infusion. On the show, cannabis expert Ry Prichard uses a 0.7 percent conversion rate to estimate the THC content of infusions. He says, "Since we aren't able to determine the effectiveness of the fat infusion, we use this estimate as the ceiling."

The next consideration is that baking or cooking with your cannabis-infused fat continues to convert acidic cannabinoid molecules to active forms, as some other THC molecules are evaporated at high temperatures. If you lab test your completed edibles, you'll usually find that some THCA remains, meaning that some molecules evaded being decarboxylated—yet another blow to the potency of your finished dish.

So, it's complicated. With this disclaimer in mind, working with cannabis at home means that you need to be open to the possibility that you might eat a little more or less THC than planned on.

Vanessa Says: A lot of thought goes into serving size when finding the right dose. For example, a salsa is a great way to increase potency in increments, much as you do with spice preferences. It's a good starting analogy for people to find their sweet spot. If a dish is something you know people will chow down on, then a lighter dose or nonpsychoactive CBD is best. Sometimes it's fun to use weed as a flavor element, even if it doesn't get you high. When Cat Cora visited the show, we had a lot of fun cooking up the leaves. They're tasty fried, candied, or even chopped up into a quick salsa verde.

THC Dosing for the Home Cook

The two big questions when you're dosing: (1) How big is a serving? (2) How much THC should each serving contain?

Working backward, you can determine that if you're baking a dozen cupcakes, and you think each guest will eat one, and your guests are newish to eating weed, you might aim for a dose of 10 milligrams of THC per cupcake. That means you'll need 120 milligrams of THC in the form of weed-infused butter for adding to the cupcake batter.

Assume you get a conversion rate of 70 percent when making your infused butter. The 120 milligrams of THC you need for the cupcake batter is 70 percent of 171.5 milligrams total THCA (51.5 milligrams are lost or destroyed during the infusion process). If you have access to cannabis flower that lab tests at 15 percent THCA, you'll

Conversion of THC in Decarboxylated Cannabis Flowers to THC Content of Infused Butter
Based on an Infusion of 3 Grams Cannabis into 8 Ounces Butter (estimated)

Amount of THC per 1 gram of decarboxylated cannabis flower	Amount of THC when multiplied by 3 grams of cannabis going into infusion	Amount of THC lost during infusion process (30 percent)	Amount of THC infused into 8 ounces of butter	Amount of THC per 1 tablespoon butter
35 mg	105 mg	31.5 mg	73.5 mg	4.5 mg
70 mg	210 mg	63 mg	147 mg	9.2 mg
105 mg	315 mg	94.5 mg	220.5 mg	13.8 mg
140 mg	420 mg	126 mg	294 mg	18.4 mg

need 1.2 grams cannabis flower for infusing into the amount of butter called for in the cupcake recipe.

While your cupcakes are baking, a small amount of THC will be lost due to oven heat. But you can still estimate that each cupcake will have at most 10 milligrams THC, and not worry if that estimate proves a little high.

In the recipes in this book, we've used lab-tested infusions, so we're able to get into the ballpark of dosing THC correctly. But variations will exist because of the potency of your starting material. We used Forbidden Fruit cannabis flower that tested at 9.05 percent THC and Forbidden Fruit trim that tested at 3.68 percent THC in their cured forms before being decarboxylated. Your weed might be more or less potent. We chose this strain because we wanted to keep the dosing low per serving.

Conversion of THCA in Cannabis Flowers to Decarboxylated THC Content Based on 1 Gram Cannabis (estimated)

Percentage of THCA per 1 gram of cannabis flower	THC in milligrams per 1 gram after decarboxylation
5	35
10	70
15	105
20	140

DO THE MATH

Following these steps will help you estimate the THC content of your infusions.

1. Starting with lab-tested cannabis that comes with a THCA percentage, determine the remaining THC content in milligrams per 1 gram after decarboxylation, assuming a 70 percent conversion rate of THCA to THC.

2. Multiply the THC content by however many grams of cannabis you are using to make your infusion. For example, we used 3 grams.

3. Subtract 30 percent of the total THC, assuming that is the amount lost during the infusion process. The remaining THC is the total estimated amount present in the infusion.

4. Divide the total amount of THC by the tablespoons of butter used (16 tablespoons in our example) to determine the estimated amount of THC in milligrams per 1 tablespoon of the infusion.

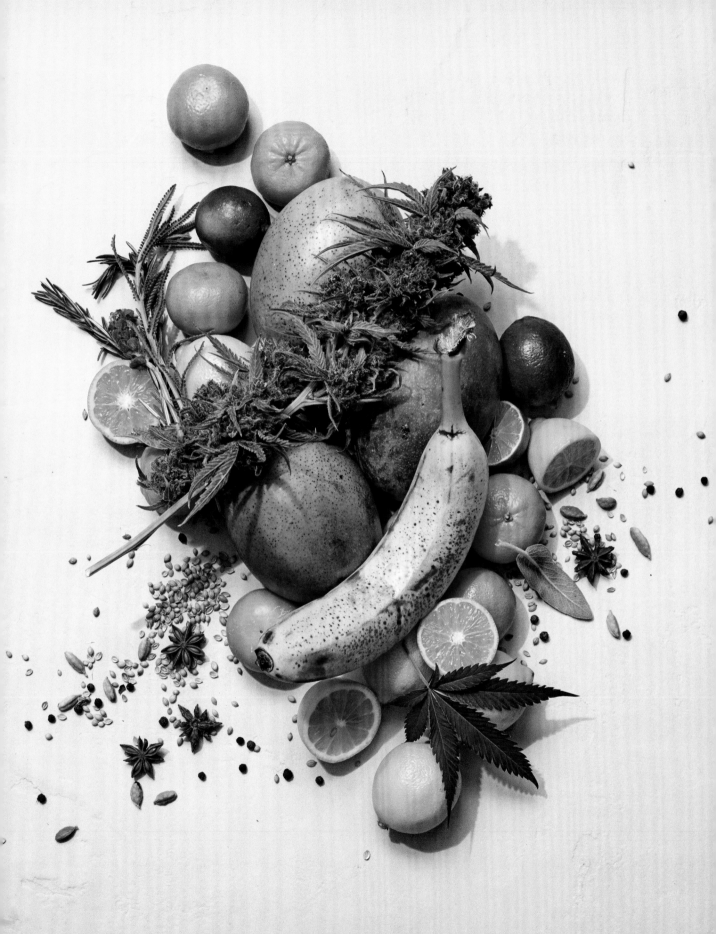

Flavors

Cooking with cannabis is about more than getting high—there's a world of flavor to explore as well. Here's what you need to know to pair cannabis strains with different foods based on how they taste and smell.

Understanding Terpenes

If you hang out with people who are seriously into dabbing, you're likely to hear the word *terpene*, or *terp* for short—a lot. It's evolved into slang for anything that tastes flavorful or awesome. The obsession with terpenes happened as cannabis connoisseurs shifted from focusing solely on potency as the primary consideration to seeing taste and aroma in a more central role—echoing the world of fine wine and craft beer. After all, any halfway decent sample of cannabis will get you high, but not every bud tastes like a ripe Meyer lemon or smells like a pine forest.

Also, back in the black-market days, cannabis strains were bred exclusively by growers looking for mind-melting psychoactivity. But it turns out that when given options, many of us actually prefer a less-intense high. Weed with THC levels at 25 percent or more packs a powerful punch. But there are plenty of consumers who will actually choose a less-potent strain with around 15 percent THC if it has a fantastic citrus taste. This is similar to the world of fine wine, where oenophiles, rather than seeking out the bottle with the highest alcohol content, look for the wine that tastes great and complements their meal.

What all this means is that the focus has now moved away from getting as wasted as possible to a more refined appreciation of the plant's diverse range of flavors and aromas. This is great news for our purposes, as it means when approaching a recipe we can source specific strains of cannabis with terpene profiles that complement what we're making.

Vanessa Says: Whenever we use terpenes—the fragrant oils of cannabis varieties—they go into a cold dish. They are volatile at high temperatures, potent in flavor, and are used much like any other culinary extract—sparingly.

What's a Terpene?

Terpenes are one of the major chemical constituents of essential oils. Scientifically known as isoprenoids, terpenes do more than just add amazing smells to cannabis. There's increasing evidence these small molecules work together with cannabinoids to increase the plant's overall healing potential, a phenomenon articulated by leading researcher Dr. Ethan Russo as the "entourage effect."

Developing and preserving high levels of terpenes in cannabis depend on how the cannabis was cultivated and processed. The growing medium, the amount of time the plant spent flowering, and whether or not it was cured properly all have a profound effect on the finished product. In other words, strains start out from seed or clone with a fixed potential to develop certain terpenes, and then the growing conditions and curing method determine to what extent those potentialities are expressed. Terpenes are composed of oil and alcohol, so the more terpenes in a concentrate, the softer and more fluid it is, with extracts such as sauce appearing less viscous due to a high terpene content.

More than 60 percent of the terpene content of a plant is lost during the drying process. This fact has led hash makers to seek out new proprietary methods of extraction that use frozen fresh cannabis, rather than dried cured flowers, as a starting ingredient. Called "live resin," this school of extract artistry is focused on preserving as many terpenes as possible.

Working with the Flavor of Cannabis

Anyone who has ever popped the top on a jar of good weed knows the distinctive, pungent scent of cannabis—a combination of intensely floral, sour, and fruity aromas that is wholly unique unto itself but with a million variations. For example, there's Zkittlez, a strain that smells like a trademarked fruity candy. Or Sour Diesel, which reminds you of a splash of spilled gasoline next to a cheese shop. There are even such grossly named strains as Cat Piss, redolent of a sharp tang of ammonia shoved under your nose.

For many years, cannabis cooks focused on covering up the taste of weed because most people don't enjoy the intense grassy flavor. Greater availability of hash and extracts have made the green taste from chlorophyll much less pronounced and therefore more appealing, however, and two schools of thought have now emerged in regard to the taste of cannabis. Some people still prefer not to have even a hint of cannabis flavor, especially when adding a psychoactive spin to a delicate recipe or a basic ingredient such as butter or oil. Seeking to minimize flavor has led to new infusion techniques involving blanching, as well as to the development of tasteless, dehydrated, powdered forms of water-soluble THC and flavorless, terpene-free extractions, such as distillate, that are used by many edible manufacturers. In the other camp, you'll find those who acknowledge weed is an acquired taste but have come to enjoy when a high-quality cannabis ingredient is thoughtfully incorporated into a dish. A slight "weed taste" is also a good way to remind yourself with every bite that "Hey, you're gonna get high," which will hopefully prevent overindulgence. The access to products such as terpenes and high-terpene extracts gives chefs an entirely new pantry of flavor possibilities to pair or contrast with in interesting ways.

Working with the diverse flavors of cannabis strains, rather than seeking to cover them up, is also a product of having access to increasingly luxurious cannabis-based ingredients. The flavor of well-made hash is pleasant, earthy, and deeply spicy, adding a rich flavor to dishes that actually elevates the finished product. Flowers, trim, and leaves still often have a strong chlorophyll taste, but you can control it by preparing them in different ways, such as frying or steeping like tea.

Vanessa Says: When planning a cannabis dinner party, you have more variables to consider. A predinner smokable is a fun way to break the ice. (Personally, I like a joint of Girl Scout Cookies.) A microdosed *amuse-bouche* (bite-size hors d'œuvre) or any finger food is good for whetting the appetite. Usually there is a main starch, such as rice or pasta. People pile these dishes on their plate, so use a lighter dose, or, better yet, a CBD option. More potent sauces are fun because guests can add as they please. It's polite to offer several dosing options. For dessert, well, sweets are the OG edible.

How to Taste and Pair Food with Cannabis

On *Bong Appétit*, cannabis expert Ry Prichard works with the guest chefs to dose each of the recipes. When asked about guidelines on pairing weed with food, he says that, perhaps more than any other plant in existence, cannabis has a chameleon-like ability to present itself with almost any scent and flavor found in nature.

Cannabis can smell uncannily like oranges or lemons, it can smell like flowers, it can smell like a dead skunk, it can even smell like lavender-thyme cookies dipped in gasoline. Really, the possibilities are endless thanks to its tendency for genetic variation and its incredibly high essential-oil content.

The way a particular cannabis strain smells is most heavily influenced by its genetics, with the mother and father plants each imparting their signature scent to the next generation in different combinations. If a breeder marries a sweet-smelling plant with a sharp, acrid-smelling one, the resulting seed plants will exist along a spectrum, with some being fully sweet, some being fully acrid, and every variation in between. So even within one "strain," such as Super Silver Haze, you may see a wide diversity of smells and flavors, each presenting a unique opportunity to pair (or contrast) with food and beverage.

Cannabis flavors, like those found in wine, beer, and food, are the result of molecules that react with your taste buds, nasal cavities, and brain to produce taste sensations. In the case of cannabis, these are largely the result of terpenes and flavonoids, which are the aromatic essential oils that, along with the cannabinoids, fill the heads of the trichome glands covering the plant and providing its unique profile. Similarly, like the flavors found in wine, beer, and food, it's useful to come up with terms to describe them. Sometimes when tasting cannabis, it's possible to pick up very distinct and specific essence notes (e.g., blueberry muffin, tennis-ball canister, lemon peel); other times, the flavors blend in such a harmonious way that it is more of a blanket category description, for example: herby, sharp, acrid, sweet, tangy, citrusy, or floral. These umbrella terms help to categorize and describe strains, but within those categories you'll find a huge number of subtleties and new combinations of flavors that were never thought possible.

One of the most exciting elements of cannabis, in a culinary sense, is its ability to interface with food and drink in very interesting and powerful ways. Much like a dry, acidic, citrus-forward rosé is the perfect partner to a piece of seared fish, the uncanny citrus qualities of Tangie, for example, complement a ponzu-soaked piece of sashimi. Today's modern cannabis products, such as separated terpenes, can give you incredible versatility, creating a rich dining experience as aroma and flavor notes bounce back and forth. While you are able to impart some complementary or contrasting flavors with infusion methods that use lower heat (such as the jar method in chapter 1), or by adding terpenes directly to food, you can also have great success pairing cannabis flavors with food via smoked or vaporized cannabis, specifically high-terpene concentrates. And, unlike alcohol, cannabis's ability to bring the user up or down with its different effects gives it an additional layer of experience, so a cannabis sommelier can start a meal with an uplifting, bright variety and end it with a rich, relaxing one.

When planning a cannabis-pairing dinner, think about the strongest flavor elements in the food and try to play off of those. Often, the most intense element is not the main protein or starch but rather a sauce or herbal component of a dish that makes it unique. Try to think about contrasting flavors as much as complementary ones; it's not always about picking something that tastes similar or goes with the dish in a conventional sense. An intriguing pairing can surprise guests and make them appreciate both the food and the cannabis more than they would have either on its own. To help you get started with understanding the ways to pair and contrast with cannabis, following are some of the most common scent and flavor categories that you'll come across.

Acrid

One function of terpenes is to deter predators from eating or otherwise damaging the plants. To do this, sometimes certain varieties will emit a smell that can be described as foul or overwhelming. Over the last decade, connoisseurs have tended to seek out these varieties, with the incredibly pungent, sharp scents cutting right through the overmatched plastic bag or jar attempting to keep them at bay. Known as "gassy" or "sour," these flavors can include elements of kerosene, glue, skunk, tires, rubber, and bad breath. While smoking something that smells like the old tennis balls in your grandpa's attic may not seem like an activity you want to do, these varieties also tend to be some of the most potent and unique, often with hordes of fans obsessing over their subtle differences. Pairing a gassy strain can be difficult, but these tend to do best with dishes that will stand up to them, such as smoked meats and herb-forward sauces (think chimichurri), but they also go suspiciously well with coffee.

Some of the most notorious gassy, acrid varieties are Chemdog, Gorilla Glue, Headband, any OG Kush variety, Sour Diesel, and Triangle Kush.

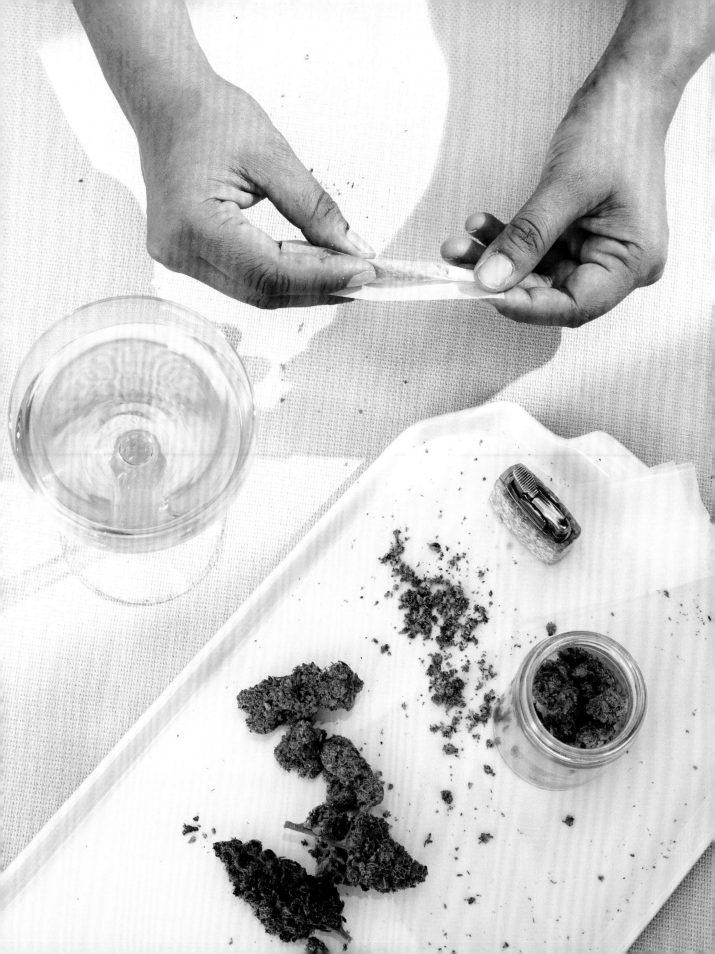

Citrusy

While other flavor categories often have hints of citrus in the mix, there are some strains that have such a strong and uncanny citrus aroma that it's at times hard to distinguish them from the real thing. The presence of limonene (which is found in grapefruit, lime, and lemon oils) is generally the reason a strain smells citrusy, but whether they smell like sweet lemon candy or garlic and lemon depends on the specific ratio and combination of other terpenes present. Citrusy varieties tend to be mentally uplifting and physically invigorating just like limonene itself, which makes sense because you more commonly find citrus-heavy flavors in strains that have traditionally been described as sativa. To pair most effectively with citrus varieties, think about how you'd use citrus in cooking; it's usually best to help brighten up a dish or add a lasting aftertaste that lingers on the palate.

Some varietals that exhibit a citrus-dominant aroma and flavor are Grapefruit, Jack's Cleaner, Jilly Bean, Lemon Diesel, Lemon G-13, Lemon Tree, Orange Cookies, Papaya, Soma's New York City Diesel (NYCD), and Tangie.

Vanessa Says: In the kitchen, we follow our nose. If a variety has more pronounced lemon notes, it might work well with fish or in a shortbread cookie. That's where the culinary side of cooking with cannabis comes in. As far as what guests choose to smoke, that's personal preference.

Earthy

Like some of the more complex and challenging wines of the world, cannabis has a whole host of rich, dank, earthy flavors present at times. *Leather*, *smoke*, *coffee*, *soil*, *peat*, and *vegetation* are some of the terms used to describe such strains, which tend to have been categorized as indicas over time. These varieties are often relaxing or sleep-inducing, perhaps due in part to the presence of terpenes such as myrcene and beta-caryophyllene, both of which are thought to have anti-anxiety properties.

Some rich and earthy varieties include Bruce Banner, Bubba Kush, Deadhead OG, Deep Chunk, Girl Scout Cookies, Hindu Kush, LA Confidential, Master Kush, Sour Bubble, and Sunset Sherbert.

Floral

Cannabis is a flower after all, so it's expected that some varieties simply smell light and fragrant like other flowers. While certain strains kick down the door to your brain like a sensory SWAT team, others lightly dance in—calming and tranquil, blending in rather than taking over. One terpene that is very common in floral varieties is linalool, which is also the most common terpene, found in lavender and many other botanicals such as bay laurel, coriander, and sweet basil. These strains can range from very soft, pleasing scents to slightly more complex, grassy ones. Floral aromas are great to use in dishes such as subtly flavored baked goods and to scent sauces and drizzles in unobtrusive ways.

Floral varieties of cannabis include Blackberry Kush, DJ Short's Flo, Grape Ape, Grape Stomper, Lavender, Purple Urkle, Strawberry Cough, and UK Cheese.

Herbal

The general flavor present in cannabis can be described as "herbal." Though this admittedly covers a huge variety of scents, they are similar in that they can be found in other herbs such as rosemary, sage, and eucalyptus, and also in things like pine trees. The most common terpenes in herbal varieties tend to be alpha-pinene, beta-pinene, beta-caryophyllene, humulene, and terpinolene, the combination of which can cover the spectrum from the tangy citrus spice of a Jack Herer to the pine-forward floral sweetness of a Maui.

Common herbal varieties include Blue Dream, Jack Herer, Malawi, Mango Haze, Maui, S.A.G.E., Super Silver Haze, and Trainwreck.

Sweet and/or Fruity

The first time you smell weed that is truly sweet, it's a life-changer. Since the odor that most casual users associate with cannabis is along the acrid, skunky side of things (because that's the way smoke usually smells), they're often totally surprised to find aromas ranging from lemon drops to cotton candy to green papaya, or a combination of ten sweet things all rolled into one. Sweet varieties usually run a spectrum from the almost creamy, neutral sugary side to the tangy, tropical fruit side, all of which offer a lot of options when it comes to pairing. Though it's tempting to pair sweet with sweet, it is often more interesting to use the sweet strains as a way to cut through something acidic or to enhance something herbal. If a strain has the distinct qualities of a specific fruit, sometimes the flavor will come through clearly enough to replace the actual fruit in a recipe, similarly to the way you can use a fruit extract.

Common strains that fit into this category include Banana Kush, Blueberry, Bubblegum, Cinderella 99, Island Sweet Skunk, Lemon Skunk, Purple Urkle, Super Lemon Haze, Vanilla Kush, and Zkittlez.

Working with Cannabis Flavors

Traditionally, most chefs of edibles have tried to hide or disguise the flavors of cannabis rather than accentuate them. While some of the subtleties of an individual strain are certainly lost during the decarboxylation and infusion processes, using lower heat (and/or less time) and utilizing more gentle methods, such as the jar method, can allow the strain's flavor to express itself more clearly in the final product. In general, the lower the heat and the less time exposed to that heat, the more terpenes and flavor are preserved. Another tip is allowing infusion mixtures to cool before opening the jar; that allows the volatile scent molecules to recondense and stay in the infusion rather than flying out at the first chance.

If you're lucky enough to have access to cannabis terpenes, they are the absolute best way to give strain-specific flavor to dishes because they come with none of the bitter or harsh flavors that can result from using other products. Putting just a single drop of quality terpenes in the bottom of a flute glass and topping with champagne will totally change the aroma and flavor of the champagne. Stirring two drops into a béchamel sauce as it cools can take its neutral creamy flavor to an entirely new place. Terpenes and other high-flavor concentrates are giving chefs a fresh toolbox of flavor possibilities that did not exist even five years ago.

Terpenes

The primary reason cannabis strains smell and taste the way they do is because of terpenes, aromatic hydrocarbons (meaning they contain only hydrogen and carbon) found in virtually every plant species. Cannabis is special because it not only carries a high concentration of terpenes in its essential oils but it also contains a very wide variety of terpenes (more than one hundred) compared to most other plants. When you smell a certain strain of weed and it reminds you of pine or lemon, it's because your nose is absorbing many of the exact same molecules as it would when smelling those things. Though certain strains are high in limonene, for example, that doesn't mean limonene is the only thing contributing to their scent—each strain is a very complex fingerprint of terpenes that enhance, balance, and cancel one another out, making it difficult at times to pinpoint what exactly you are smelling.

Beyond just smelling good (or bad), terpenes have definable physical and cerebral effects on humans, as demonstrated in ancient practices such as aromatherapy. For example, studies have shown that humans exposed to high limonene scents, such as grapefruit essential oil, often see improvement with depression, fatigue, and headaches. Now, many modern cannabis researchers believe that the complex ratios of the cannabinoids and the aroma and flavor compounds, such as the terpenes and flavonoids that exist within a strain, are what actually produces its unique effects.

So smelling that bright, tangy Durban Poison makes you happy not only because you're about to smoke it soon and get really high but the actual compounds within it help cause that reaction. In addition, the way that an individual plant is grown can increase the amount of total terpenes as well as the presence of specific ones. This means that a skilled grower using a particular type of nutrient may bring out more of the strain-centric flavor and effect of a varietal than someone who just threw a seed in the ground and fed it water. Similarly, high-terpene concentrates may provide a more directed experience than flowers and terpene-free concentrates, such as distillate and isolate, thanks to the higher amounts of these compounds. To help understand terpenes further, here is a description of the most common ones and some popular varieties of cannabis in which they can be found.

Limonene

Present predominately in sativa strains, limonene also appears in citrus rinds, rosemary, juniper, and peppermint and is a significant component of citrus-based cleaning products. Strains of cannabis that possess a bright, acidic, sweet lemon flavor are easily infused into butter or olive oil and paired with any sweet or savory dish that traditionally uses lemons. Determine whether your chosen cannabis is more sweet, sour, or tart and then pair accordingly. For example, Super Lemon Haze is a sativa that's more tart, perfect for pairing with a light sugary dessert, while a sweet Tangie would complement fish more readily, and a distinctive Sour Diesel will shine through even when paired with bold rosemary and rich lamb.

Look for Bubba Kush, Durban Poison, LA Confidential, Sour Diesel, Super Lemon Haze, and Tangie, among many others.

Linalool

Floral and spicy, linalool is found in hundreds of plants, including lavender, sweet basil, mint, laurels, birch, rosewood, and coriander, and has sedative, anti-anxiety, and stress-relieving effects. For thousands of years, lavender has been considered an effective sleep aid due to the linalool it contains. The strain Lavender is rich in linalool, works well in desserts like cake and ice cream, and can be combined with lemon to create sophisticated cocktails or elixirs.

Found in Amnesia Haze, G-13, Headband, Ingrid, LA Confidential, Lavender, and Skywalker OG, among others.

Myrcene

Present in hops, lemongrass, citrus, mangoes, verbena, bay leaves, ylang-ylang, eucalyptus, and thyme, myrcene is earthy and musky and carries a hint of clove, balsamic, and fruitiness. When creating an infusion with a myrcene-rich cannabis strain, consider the season, the mood of the occasion, and the cuisine you'd like to cook. Citrus, mango, chiles, and coconut milk work well with strains that express fruity or lemongrass terps, such as Pineapple Kush and Grand Daddy Purps. But other earthier myrcene-rich strains such as Northern Lights would pair better with richer flavors, including roasted meats, orange glazes, thyme, and goat cheese.

Found in Blue Dream, Himalayan Gold, Skunk #1, Sour Diesel, and White Widow, among many others.

Pinene

The most common terp found in cannabis, pinene is also present in conifers like pine and fir trees, as well as herbs such as rosemary, basil, parsley, dill, and sage, and is a principal component of turpentine. When using a cannabis strain high in pinene, such as Jack Herer or Island Sweet Skunk, infuse it into olive oil for a seamless integration into Mediterranean cuisine, and blend it with savory, herbaceous flavors that complement the natural taste of weed. The strong flavors of grilled meats and vegetables, garlic, and tomatoes stand up to an assertive addition of cannabis, while the richness of foods like egg yolk, mashed potatoes, and duck provide a pleasant contrast to the herb.

Found in Bubba Kush, Chemdog, Dutch Treat, Island Sweet Skunk, Jack Herer, OG Kush, Romulan, Super Silver Haze, and Trainwreck, among many others.

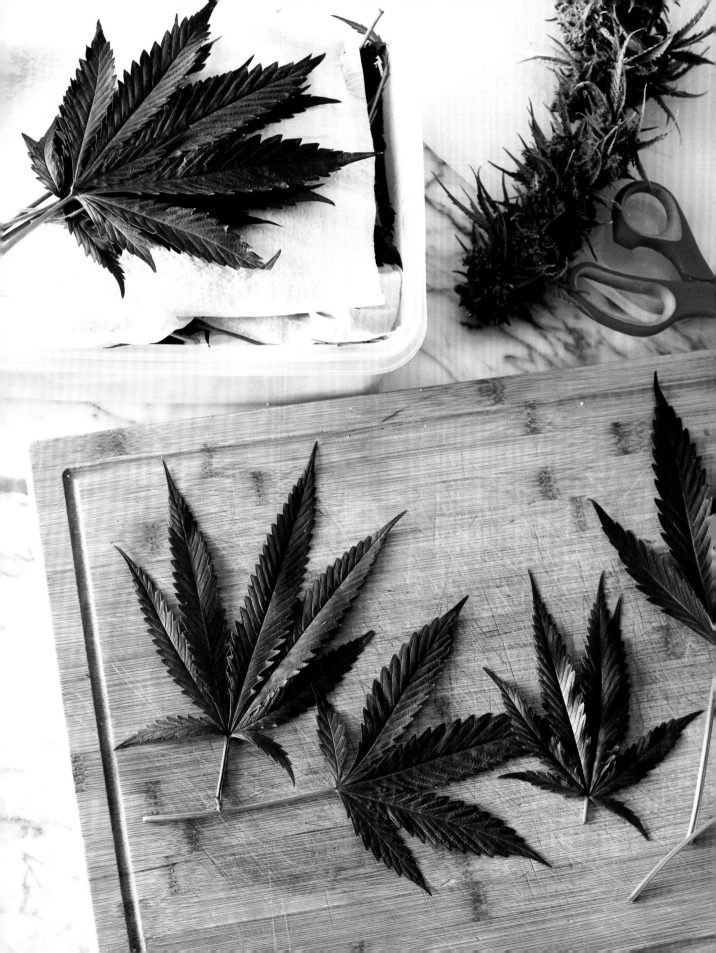

Preparing Your Weed for Cooking: Tips and Techniques

For many years, the sole goal of cooking with cannabis was to get as high as possible as efficiently as possible. Underground edibles makers traditionally focused on using less-pricey parts of the plant that aren't suitable for smoking and would otherwise go to waste, like the sugar leaves, trim, shake from the bottom of a bag, or low-quality schwag buds. Recipes from that era prioritized wringing every last particle of THC from these lesser cuts, with flavor a distant secondary consideration. So if you've ever wondered why pot food has a reputation for tasting pretty crappy, that's the reason.

In general, the more expensive a cannabis ingredient is, the better it will taste. Trim is cheap and tastes very green. Flower costs more and tastes better while still being herbaceous and vegetal, much like basil, arugula, or parsley. Precious kief, hashes, and extracts are pricier than flower and trim, but the absence of chlorophyll makes concentrates taste much better, with unique earthy, spicy flavors.

Today, with legalization changing the game, weed costs are falling while the diversity of cannabis ingredients available—a dizzying array of extracts, hashes, and flowers—is increasing exponentially. In the future, once the costs have dropped enough to make these concentrated ingredients accessible to nearly everyone, cooks will probably use kief and hash. You can eliminate the grassy taste of cannabis entirely by making your own kief, but you'll need a lot of weed to end up with even a little bit of the precious result. Yield is highly dependent on how resinous and full of trichomes the plant material is, so only a rough guesstimate is possible. If you use trim to make kief, you might yield 10 percent of the weight of the plant matter, and if you use flower, the yield might be up to 20 percent. For example, 1 pound of trim could be sifted to yield 45 grams of kief, while 1 pound of flower would be more resinous, yielding maybe 90 grams of kief.

It's easy to add a measured high to any dish if using kief. For example, 1 gram of the raw Forbidden Fruit kief we used for this book contains 44.5 milligrams of THC, enough to dose more than eight servings with 5 milligrams each. For a visual, that same gram of kief equals 1 teaspoon, so ⅛ teaspoon raw kief is sufficient to add a subtle psychoactive effect to a plate of food. Once you toast kief—decarboxylating it—that potency skyrockets, as acidic THCA converts into psychoactive THC, but the flavor will change to a much more pungent, roasted taste, losing most of its terpenes. Our raw Forbidden Fruit kief contained 4.5 percent THC but also

58.4 percent THCA, so when fully activated, it can reach up to 500 milligrams of THC per 1 gram of kief. That ⅛ teaspoon kief could now contain up to 62.5 milligrams of fully decarboxylated THC.

Making Kief

Sifting your herb through a kief box that collects THC-laden trichomes as you break up and roll your bud is a great way to passively bank some THC for a rainy day. Or, you can process your herb in a weed grinder with a kief-sorting compartment that will isolate the resin glands as you grind. With either of these methods, however, it'll take time to accumulate a decent amount of kief, which can then be sprinkled on top of a bowl, rolled into a joint, or added to recipes much like a spice. To collect larger amounts of kief quickly, you can make a dry-ice shaker (see page 57, or buy one, if you're fancy) to separate the trichomes from the plant matter.

Comparison of Decarboxylation on active THC Content of Cannabis Ingredients (Option 1)

Type of Cannabis Ingredient		Time in a 240°F oven	THC Percentage by Weight	THC Content	Acidic THC Content
Flower: Forbidden Fruit strain (dried and cured)		30 minutes	10.89	34.9 mg/g	84.2 mg/g
		60 minutes	10.75	80.3 mg/g	31 mg/g
Trim: Forbidden Fruit strain (dried and cured)		30 minutes	7.69	72.3 mg/g	5.3 mg/g
		60 minutes	6.25	61.7 mg/g	0.9 mg/g

How to Activate THC through Decarboxylation

Fresh-picked cannabis won't get you high if you eat it because the nonpsychoactive THCA found naturally in the plant has to be heated before it transforms into the version of THC that very much does get you high. This happens instantly when you smoke a joint, and over a longer period of time when you activate cannabis before infusing it into food.

Also known as *decarboxylating* in chemistry terms, this process simply means removing the carboxyl molecule found in THCA (the nonpsychoactive acidic form), thereby transforming it into the fun kind of THC. You can decarboxylate cannabis a few different ways, including quickly at a high temperature or slowly at a low temperature. "Low and slow" has been the traditional favorite, as it minimizes the risk of burning your precious pot. Keep in mind that THC boils off at 314°F, so you should never come close to that danger point. Terpenes are even more volatile, with delicate caryophyllene evaporating at 246°F, tougher linalool at 388°F, and other well-known terps disappearing at points in between.

Preserving as many cannabinoids and terpenes as possible means using a low temperature, with 240°F generally recommended for proper decarboxylation. Timing is also important, with 30 to 60 minutes typically recommended for a successful decarb. Remember, heating your cannabis for too long will result in THC converting to CBN, leaving you less high and much sleepier. Plant material with a higher moisture content will need longer to decarb than kief or hash, so keep that in mind when using an extract or hash

for cooking. And if you are pressed for time, you can crank up the temperature to 300°F and toast (bake) the plant material for 10 to 15 minutes, though you'll be losing more terpenes.

Here, we describe two different methods for decarboxylation, baking (aka toasting) and one directly inspired by sous vide cooking, in which food enclosed in a vacuum-sealed bag is immersed in a hot water bath to cook at a precise, continuous temperature for a specific amount of time. You can pick the one that best fits your time, equipment, skill level, and taste preferences. You can eat your properly decarboxylated cannabis as is (and it will get you high), combine it with a bit of melted butter or coconut oil and put into capsules, or infuse it into a basic ingredient such as butter, cream, milk, coconut oil, alcohol, or glycerin. Always begin by coarsely grinding your cannabis material to increase its surface area.

Method 1: Baking

This method is simple, but be aware that many ovens can fluctuate wildly in temperature. So before you begin, use an oven thermometer to make sure your oven is properly calibrated.

Heat the oven to 240°F.

Spread the freshly ground cannabis flower, trim, kief, or hash on a glass pie plate in an even layer and cover the plate with aluminum foil, crimping the foil around the rim to seal securely.

If your cannabis is very dry or there's not much of it, toast for 30 minutes. If the flower or trim is green and moist or if you have more than 28 grams, toast for up to 60 minutes, checking

DRYING AND CURING CANNABIS

If you grow your own backyard cannabis plants, harvest them when the flowers are at their fullest, and the trichomes, when examined under a magnifying glass, have turned from clear to a milky white. At this point, remove the fan leaves for juicing, cooking, or compost. Hang the cut flower stalks upside down in a cool, dry, dark place until they are dry and the stems can be snapped, 4 to 5 days.

The next step is to break down the plants into smaller pieces. Using a pair of small, sharp scissors, cut the flowers off the stalks and into smaller bundles of buds, removing as many stems and sugar leaves as possible. Reserve the trim for culinary purposes.

Cure the dry buds by packing them into glass canning jars and sealing for another 5 to 7 days. Uncap the jars every day and let them sit open for an hour or so, then seal again. This process allows any remaining moisture to slowly evaporate.

Test a flower after 5 days to check if it's properly cured. It should grind easily, roll nicely into a joint, and burn without going out or needing to be re-lit more than once, leaving behind a white ash. If flowers are still too wet, continue curing for a few more days before checking again.

Of course, if you're buying flower at a dispensary, all of these steps have been handled for you.

DIY Kief Shaker

Yield: 0.7 grams if using trim;
1.4 grams if using flower

After shaking out the kief, you'll still need to toast it to make it much more psychoactive. Once you've done that, it's the perfect add-in to whatever you're planning on cooking. Just like cannabis flower or trim, kief is a raw plant ingredient that needs to be heated to fully activate all the potential THC. And if you happen to have frozen your freshly harvested plants, this kief is a great way to preserve more terpenes and flavors.

Equipment

Clean 1-quart canning jar

2 cups dry ice (if using dried cannabis)

2 or 3 rubber bands

12-inch-square silk screen, 90 to 120 micron

12 by 16-inch sheet parchment paper

Small opaque glass jar with a tight lid

Metal dough scraper

7 grams trim or flower, dried and cured (see facing page) or frozen

Put the trim or flower in the canning jar; if using dried cannabis, add the dry ice. Use the rubber bands to secure the silk screen over the mouth of the jar.

Invert the jar over the parchment paper. Shake the jar vigorously to release the kief, which will be a golden blonde to tan powder, onto the paper. Stop shaking when the kief begins to show a slight green tinge. (This indicates the plant matter is beginning to break up and get into your kief.)

Transfer the kief from the parchment to the opaque jar, using the dough scraper to ease any bits still clinging to the screen into the jar. Cap the jar tightly. Store in a cool, dark place for up to 1 month (for maximum freshness) or freeze for up to 1 year.

and stirring it periodically to make sure it's not getting too brown or burned. The flowers should look toasted and smell very fragrant. If using kief or hash and working with no more than 14 grams, toast for 20 to 30 minutes. If processing more than 14 grams, toast for 45 to 60 minutes, stirring every 10 to 15 minutes, until it smells very toasty. When the kief or hash is done decarbing, it will be slightly browner than it was originally.

When the time is up, remove the pie plate from the oven and let it sit, covered, until it is cool to the touch. This step allows any vaporized cannabinoids to settle back into the plant matter. Use immediately, or transfer to an airtight glass container and store in a cool, dark place for up to 1 month.

This method can also make your weed taste toasted, which can work in some recipes but not in others.

Method 2: "Sous Vide"

Sous vide cooking is a fairly recent culinary trend in which food enclosed in a vacuum-sealed bag is immersed in a hot water bath to cook at a precise, continuous temperature for a specific amount of time. This technology is tailor-made for infusing cannabis, which requires precise temperature control to maximize the THC extraction but control the bitter flavors that can come from over-extraction. You will need an immersion circulator and, ideally, a vacuum sealer to try this method. With this method, there's not really a way to over-extract the material, so you could "set it and forget it" if you don't have 6 hours to sit by the stove.

To decarboxylate flowers, trim, kief, or hash: Vacuum seal your cannabis ingredients in a food-safe plastic bag.

Set your sous vide cooker to 200°F.

Immerse the sealed bag in the hot water and allow it to simmer for 4 to 6 hours. Simmer longer for larger quantities.

To make infusions: In a food-safe plastic bag, combine decarboxylated cannabis with melted butter, oil, or glycerin.

Vaccum seal the bag, immerse in the hot water, and allow it to simmer for 4 to 6 hours. Simmer longer for larger quantities.

Whether you choose to add that extra toasting step really depends on how high you want to get. If you're looking for a low dose, you can skip it. If you want to get as high as possible, definitely do it and then go directly to infusing your weed into a chosen fat, as decarboxylation before infusing is still the best way to fully activate all of the potential THC. If you want to rely on the heat of infusion to activate the THC, that's fine. It's just not as efficient.

IS DECARBOXYLATION NECESSARY?

Decarboxylation of cannabis is necessary if you want to get really fucking high. If you don't mind using more weed to get less high, you can skip the whole process and activate the THC in your cannabis during the infusion process. The results will still be psychoactive, but there will be significant unconverted THCA remaining in the herb, so it won't be as psychoactive as it could be.

Comparison of Decarboxylation on THC Content of Cannabis Ingredients: Flower and Trim after 30 Minutes and 60 Minutes at 240°F

Type of Cannabis Ingredient	Oven Time at 240°F	THC Percentage by Weight	THC Content	Acidic THC Content
Flower: Forbidden Fruit strain (dried and cured)	30 minutes	10.89	34.9 mg/g	84.2 mg/g
Trim: Forbidden Fruit strain (dried and cured)	30 minutes	7.69	72.3 mg/g	5.3 mg/g
Flower: Forbidden Fruit strain (dried and cured)	60 minutes	10.75	80 mg/g	31 mg/g
Trim: Forbidden Fruit strain (dried and cured)	60 minutes	6.25	61.7 mg/g	0.9 mg/g

As you can see, 60 minutes at 240°F is plenty of time to activate almost all of the THCA in your flower or trim and convert it to THC. The THC percentage does begin to drop, however, because some cannabinoids are evaporating.

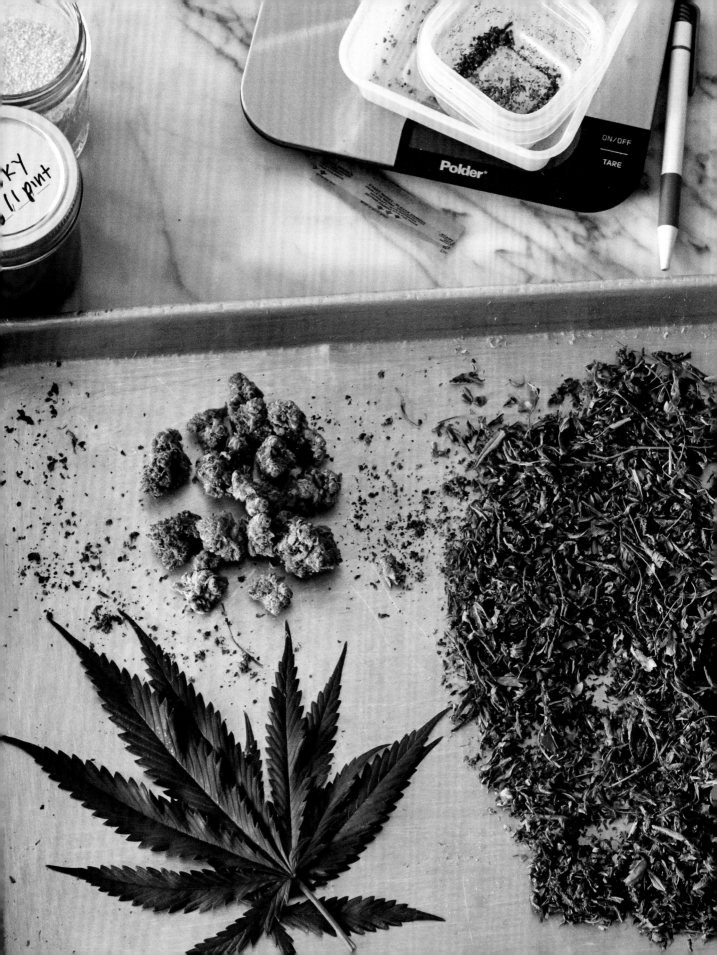

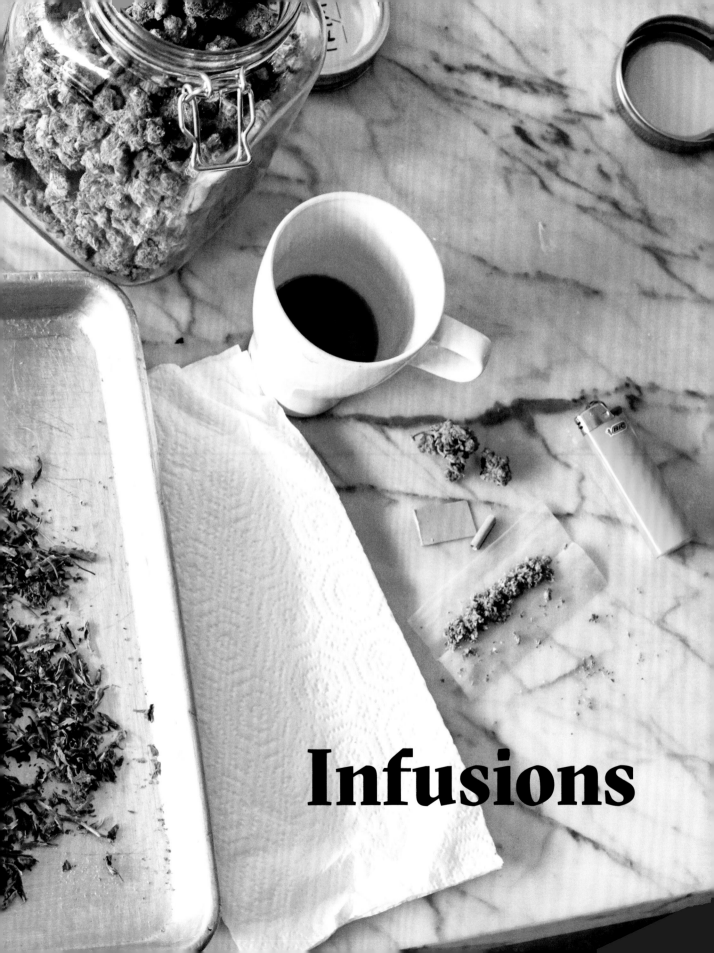

Infusions

There are many different methods for infusing cannabis into fats, suitable for every skill level and tailored to fit various equipment modalities. But they all seek to accomplish the same goal: removing cannabinoids from the plant matter and transferring those precious molecules as efficiently as possible into the chosen fat.

Why Fats?

Cannabinoids are hydrophobic, meaning they hate water. But they have a fetish for lipids, gravitating toward fats whenever possible. For this reason, the most effective cannabis infusions use fats, including butter, oil, lard, schmaltz, cream, and milk. Absorbing cannabis into your body along with fat also makes it more bioavailable, meaning it feels more potent in your body, versus eating the same amount of decarboxylated cannabis without the accompanying fat.

When it comes to the best fats to use, saturated fats that are solid at room temperature—butter, coconut oil, lard—seem to absorb more cannabinoids than liquid fats, such as oils, though the difference is negligible. Butter, oil, pancetta fat, heavy cream, cow's milk, and coconut milk all work to get THC into food. Adding sugar has the effect of making THC seem more potent, hence the longtime association of weed food with sweets.

On their own, sugar and glycerin aren't great mediums for infusions, which is why we infuse cannabis into fat before combining it with honey. Alcohol does a good job of attracting cannabinoids and preserving them, but it's not as good as fat.

On the show, when Ry seeks to introduce cannabinoids to recipes that don't call for fat, he turns to modern extracts like activated isolates and distillates, as they dissolve easily into foods. Relatively new to the marketplace is water-soluble THC, a product of chemical tweaking that is primarily used for adding cannabis to products like drinks.

Vanessa Says: Hands down, my favorite part of throwing a cannabis dinner party is cooking up new ideas in the kitchen. Any dish can have cannabis in it as long as there is fat or alcohol. The challenge is to come up with new techniques. When Debbie Michail cold-smoked labneh, or Louis Tikaram smashed fried cannabis nugs into his Thai dressing, sparks went off. I remember the first time I tasted a cannabis fan leaf and thought, "Yum! This tastes like shiso!"

Squeezing all the infused oil out of the plant matter improves your yield.

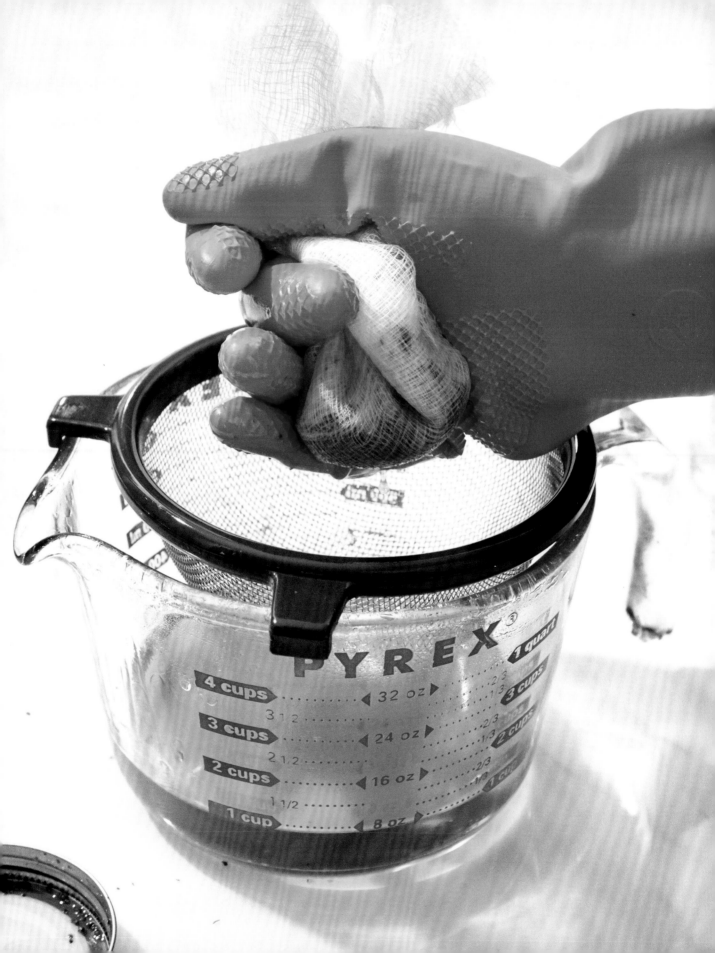

Weed-Infused Oil

MUNCHIES Test Kitchen

Yield: ¾ cup

	THC IN MILLIGRAMS	
	Flower-Infused Oil	Kief-Infused Oil
1 tsp	3.5	2.8
1 Tbsp	10.4	8.4
¼ cup	41.6	33.6
½ cup	83.2	67.2
¾ cup	124.8	100

This is the simplest, easiest way to get weed into food and then into yourself. It's a neat and clean method of infusing different oils simultaneously. Plus, it keeps the smells contained, for those of you with less-chill neighbors.

You can infuse cannabis into any type of oil. We typically use infused olive oil in salad dressings, marinades, and salsas; our infused canola is in a dipping sauce that accompanies pork wontons (see page 108); and infused coconut oil goes into the Strawberry "Cheesecake" on page 205 and the whipped honey on page 74.

Infusing raw kief into olive oil won't return the most potent oil, but the oil will be subtle and nicely flavored, making it appropriate for use in recipes where simple flavors would be overwhelmed by a grassy cannabis taste. Drizzle it over fresh pasta or the focaccia on page 223. Use a flower-infused olive oil for the tomato salad on page 120 or the *panzanella*-inspired salad on page 123, where the flavors complement the grassy taste of this oil, which is easy to dose at 10 milligrams THC per 1 tablespoon.

You can infuse a number of different oils simultaneously with this method, which keeps each oil in its own canning jar. (Label the top of each jar to avoid confusion.) If you are infusing coconut oil, you will need to melt it first, as it is solid at room temperature.

Equipment

12-ounce canning jar with lid

Stockpot

Kitchen towel

Silicone oven mitt or jar tongs

Mesh strainer

Cheesecloth

Liquid measuring cup

1 cup oil; such as olive, coconut, grapeseed, or canola

3 grams cannabis flower or 1 gram raw kief

Vanessa Says: For the basic infusion of flower into fat, you'll find plenty of information about decarboxylation, or heating cannabis to release carboxylic acid and activate the flower before infusing it into fat. I am more concerned with how long the flower is infused into fat. The longer a plant is steeped in fat, the more bitter green flavor will be pulled.

Pour the oil into the canning jar. Add the cannabis material and stir to combine. Seal the jar tightly.

Stand the jar upright in the stockpot and add water until it is level with the top of the jar. Place the stockpot, uncovered, over high heat and bring to a low boil. Let boil for 2 hours, checking the water every now and again and adding more as needed to maintain the original level. After the first hour, "burp" the jar by unsealing the lid to release any pressure buildup and then recap it.

After 2 hours, lay the kitchen towel on a heatproof work surface. Using the oven mitt, remove the jar from the water, set it on the towel, and let cool until it can be handled. Then, while the oil is still liquid, line the strainer with the cheesecloth and strain the oil into the measuring cup, squeezing any solids at the very end to extract all of the fat. Compost or discard the plant matter. If you used kief, there's no need to strain.

Use right away, or transfer to a clean jar and store in the refrigerator or freezer for up to 3 months.

Pro Tip: An infused oil made with kief will taste better than one made with flower. We used raw kief for this infusion. For a big potency boost, decarboxylate your kief by toasting in a 240°F oven for 30 minutes before infusing.

Comparison of THC Content of Olive Oil Infused with Decarboxylated Flower and Raw Kief

Type of Cannabis Ingredient	Amount of Each Infusion Ingredient	Activated THC	THC Content	Acidic THC Content
Flower: Forbidden Fruit strain (toasted for 60 minutes to decarb)	3 g flower in 1 cup olive oil	10.4 mg per 1 Tbsp	0.8 mg/g 0.7 mg/ml	0.3 mg/g 0.3 mg/ml
Kief: Forbidden Fruit strain (raw)	1 g kief in 1 cup olive oil	8.4 mg per 1 Tbsp	0.6 mg/g 0.6 mg/ml	2.3 mg/g 2.2 mg/ml

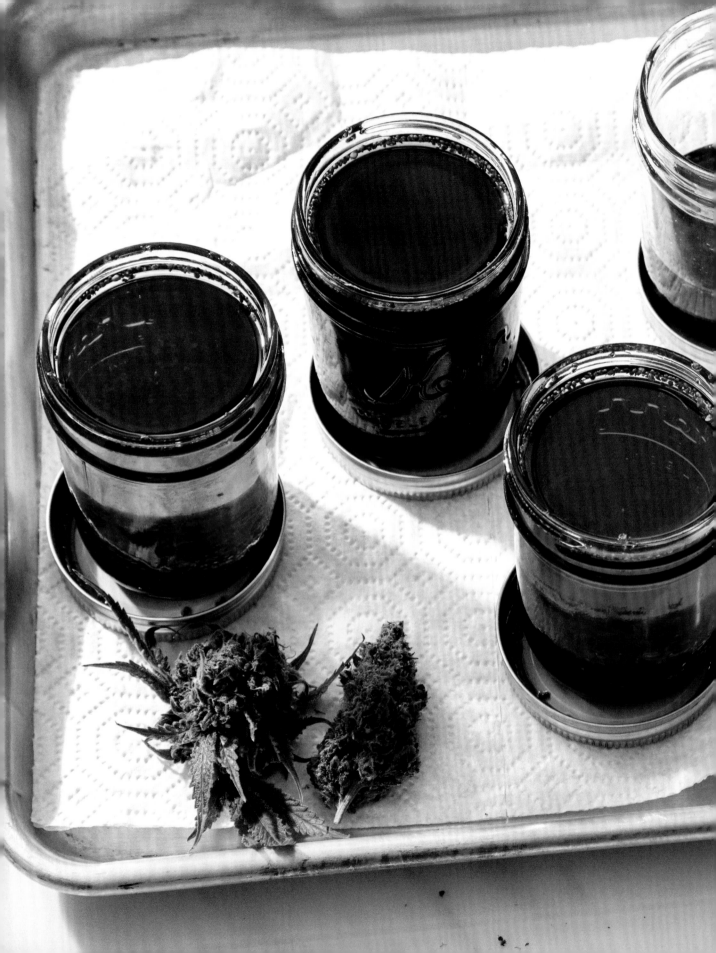

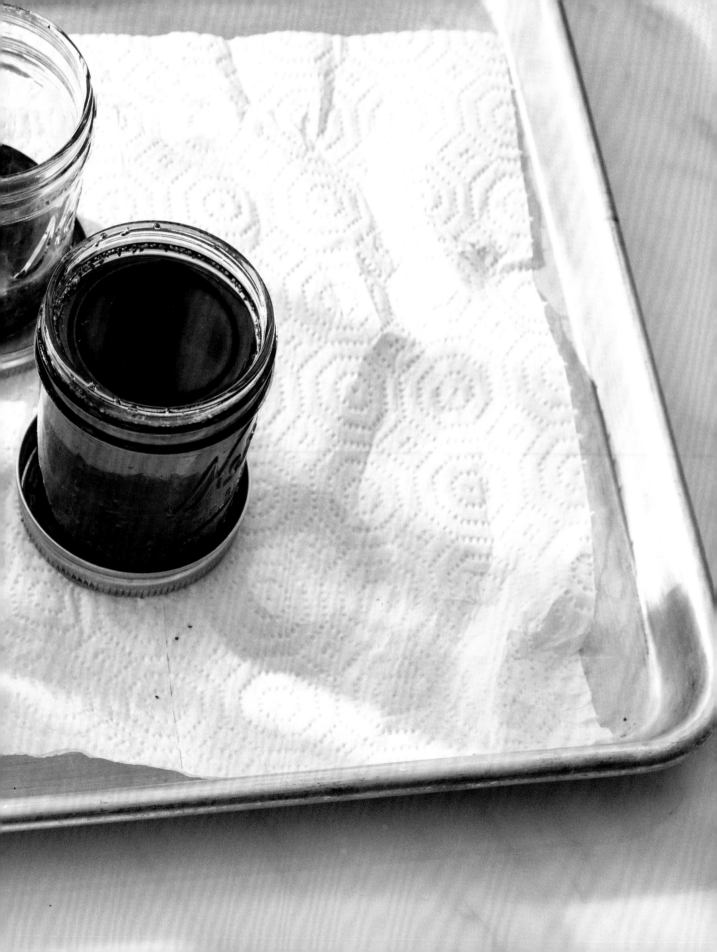

Weed-Infused Butter

MUNCHIES Test Kitchen

Yield: ¾ cup

	THC IN MILLIGRAMS	
	Flower-Infused Butter	Kief-Infused Butter
1 tsp	5.5	2
1 Tbsp	16.7	6
¼ cup	66.8	24
½ cup	133.6	48
¾ cup	200	72

You use the same method to infuse butter that you use to infuse oil. For the most efficient infusion, purchase European-style butter, which has a higher butterfat content than conventional butter. We store the finished butter in a jar, but you can also freeze it in an ice-cube tray, which makes it easy to measure consistent doses.

Although the infusion process doesn't do much to activate the THC in kief, we find that butter infused with kief tastes the best, making it perfect for diners seeking a low THC dose with excellent flavor. It is ideal for simple applications that call for larger amounts of butter, such as drizzling over popcorn or spreading on a piece of toasted rustic bread. The flower-infused butter works well for baking, as it has relatively low potency and a pleasant but distinct cannabis flavor. Use it in the brownies for the sundae on page 195 or in the Adult Celebration Cake on page 211.

12-ounce canning jar with lid

Stockpot

Kitchen towel

Silicone oven mitt or jar tongs

Mesh strainer

Cheesecloth

Liquid measuring cup

1 cup unsalted European-style butter, melted

3 grams cannabis flower or 1 gram raw kief

Pour the butter into the canning jar. Add the cannabis material and stir to combine. Seal the jar tightly.

Stand the jar upright in the stockpot and add water until it is level with the top of the jar. Place the stockpot, uncovered, over high heat and bring to a gentle simmer. Let simmer for 2 hours, checking the water every now and again and adding more as needed to maintain the original level. Make sure it never reaches a full boil. After the first hour, "burp" the jar by unsealing the lid to release any pressure buildup and then recap it.

After 2 hours, lay the kitchen towel on a heatproof work surface. Using the oven mitt, remove the jar from the water, set it on the towel, and let cool until it can be handled. Then, while the butter is still liquid, line the strainer with the cheesecloth and strain the butter into the measuring cup, squeezing any solids at the very end to extract all of the butter. Compost or discard the plant matter. If you used kief, you don't need to strain.

Use right away, or transfer to a clean jar and store in the refrigerator for up to 2 weeks or in the freezer for up to 3 months.

Comparison of THC Content of Butter Infused with Decarboxylated Flower and Raw Kief

Type of Cannabis Ingredient	Amount of Infusion Ingredients	Activated THC	THC Content	Acidic THC Content
Flower: Forbidden Fruit strain (toasted for 60 minutes to decarb)	3 g flower in 1 cup melted butter	16.7 mg per 1 Tbsp	1.2 mg/g	0.5 mg/g
Kief: Forbidden Fruit strain (raw)	1 g kief in 1 cup melted butter	6.1 mg per 1 Tbsp	0.4 mg/g	2.9 mg/g

Weed-Infused Brown Butter

MUNCHIES Test Kitchen
Yield: ¾ cup

0.5 gram raw kief

¾ cup unsalted butter, cut into 1-tablespoon pieces

	THC IN MILLIGRAMS
1 tsp	2.9
1 Tbsp	8.8
¼ cup	35.2
½ cup	70.4
¾ cup	106

Nutty, toasty brown butter is good over the gnocchi on page 141 or in the chocolate chip cookies on page 196. Its earthy, umami flavor is only improved with the addition of raw kief. Making brown butter is easy, but you do have to pay attention so it doesn't burn, which would be a major bummer if you've already poured it over a bunch of kief.

Put the kief in a small heatproof bowl.

In a sauté pan over medium heat, melt the butter, stirring constantly. The butter will melt, then begin to bubble and foam. When the foam starts to subside, the milk solids will begin to brown and the butter will smell nutty. Keep stirring for just a second, then pour the brown butter over the kief and stir to dissolve.

Let the butter cool and set before using, or transfer to a clean jar, let cool, cover, and store in the refrigerator for up to 3 days or in the freezer for up to 6 months.

Pro Tip: You can increase the potency of this brown butter by decarboxylating the kief. Place it in a ramekin, cover the ramekin tightly with aluminum foil, and toast in a 240°F oven for 15 minutes. We were surprised to see the weed-infused brown butter return a higher lab test result than regular infused butter—it's probably because the super-fast infusion preserves more cannabinoids.

Weed-Infused Coconut Milk

MUNCHIES Test Kitchen

Yield: 1 cup

Equipment

Double boiler

Mesh strainer

Cheesecloth

Liquid measuring cup

7 grams cannabis trim, ground and decarboxylated (see page 55)

1 cup coconut milk

	THC IN MILLIGRAMS
1 tsp	1.9
1 Tbsp	5.9
¼ cup	23.6
½ cup	47.2
¾ cup	70.8
1 cup	93.6

Infusing coconut milk is a great option for vegan dishes, along with a variety of curries and Thai or Indian soups and stews. We used infused coconut milk in the moqueca on page 183 and the crab gratin on page 114.

Set up the double boiler and bring the water to a simmer. Combine the trim and coconut milk in the top of the double boiler and cook, stirring occasionally, for 30 minutes. Remove from the heat and let cool.

Line the strainer with the cheesecloth and strain the coconut milk into the measuring cup, squeezing the solids at the very end to extract all of the coconut milk. Compost or discard the plant matter.

Use right away, or transfer to a clean jar and store in the refrigerator for up to 4 days.

Weed-Infused Cream

MUNCHIES Test Kitchen

Yield: 1 cup

	THC IN MILLIGRAMS
1 tsp	11
1 Tbsp	33.5
¼ cup	134
½ cup	268
¾ cup	402
1 cup	535

Equipment

Double boiler

Mesh strainer

Cheesecloth

Liquid measuring cup

7 grams cannabis trim, ground and decarboxylated (see page 55)

1 cup heavy cream

Always use the best organic, full-fat cream you can find so there are enough lipids to support a potent cannabis infusion. Nondairy creams can also be infused using this method, especially coconut cream, which has a high fat content. For milk alternatives made from almond, hemp, or soy, the fat content must be 4 grams per serving, at the very least, or you're just wasting weed.

Use this infused cream to create the ricotta on page 233, the ice cream on page 193, the nacho sauce on page 99, or the filling for the Adult Celebration Cake on page 211.

Set up the double boiler and bring the water to a simmer. Combine the trim and cream in the top of the double boiler and cook, stirring occasionally, for 30 minutes. Remove from the heat and let cool.

Line the strainer with the cheesecloth and strain the cream into the measuring cup, squeezing the solids at the very end to extract all of the cream. Compost or discard the plant matter.

Use right away, or transfer to a clean jar and store in the refrigerator for up to 4 days.

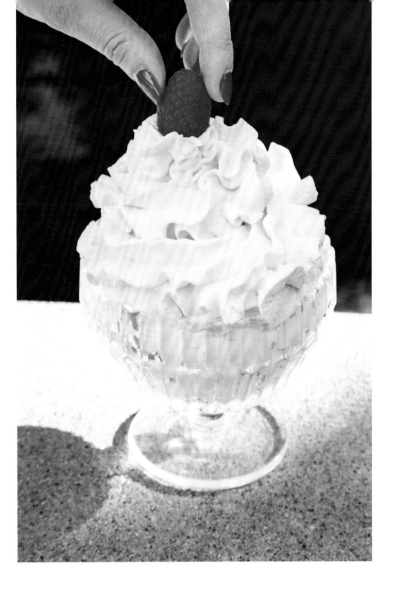

Whipped Weed-Infused Cream

¼ cup weed-infused cream (see facing page)

¼ cup heavy cream

1 tablespoon confectioners' sugar

½ teaspoon vanilla extract

In a large bowl, combine the infused cream, heavy cream, confectioners' sugar, and vanilla. Using a whisk or handheld blender, beat until stiff peaks form. Keep refrigerated for up to 2 days; rewhip if it looks deflated.

Whipped Weed-Infused Honey or Syrup

MUNCHIES Test Kitchen

Yield: ¾ cup

	THC IN MILLIGRAMS
1 tsp	1.5
1 Tbsp	4.7
¼ cup	18.8
½ cup	37.6
¾ cup	56

Equipment

16-ounce canning jar with lid

Stockpot

Kitchen towel

Silicone oven mitt or jar tongs

Blender

Squeeze bottle

¾ cup honey

2 tablespoons MCT coconut oil

0.5 gram kief

When you buy weed honey at a dispensary, chances are it's made by simply mixing a viscous cannabis concentrate extract directly into honey, resulting in a product with little bioavailability. This honey is simple to make, and it is effective because of the addition of oil as fat. It's important to use medium chain triglycerides (MCT) oil, which is a type of coconut oil that is liquid at room temperature. Otherwise your honey will solidify at cooler temperatures and be difficult to pour.

Use this honey in the peanut butter on page 232 and in the Adult Celebration Cake on page 211. You can also stir it directly into a cup of tea or drizzle it over ice cream. This same method can be used with molasses, agave nectar, or maple syrup.

Pour the honey and coconut oil into the canning jar, add the kief, and stir to combine. Seal the jar tightly.

Stand the jar upright in the stockpot and add water until it is level with the top of the jar. Place the stockpot, uncovered, over high heat and bring to a boil. Lower the heat and let simmer for 2 hours, checking the water every now and again and adding more as needed to maintain the original level.

After 2 hours, lay the kitchen towel on a heatproof work surface. Using the oven mitt, remove the jar from the water, set it on the towel, and let cool until it can be handled. Then, pour the infused honey into the blender and blend on high speed until the mixture is emulsified, 3 to 5 minutes.

Transfer the honey to the squeeze bottle for easy access and store in a cool, dark place for up to 6 months.

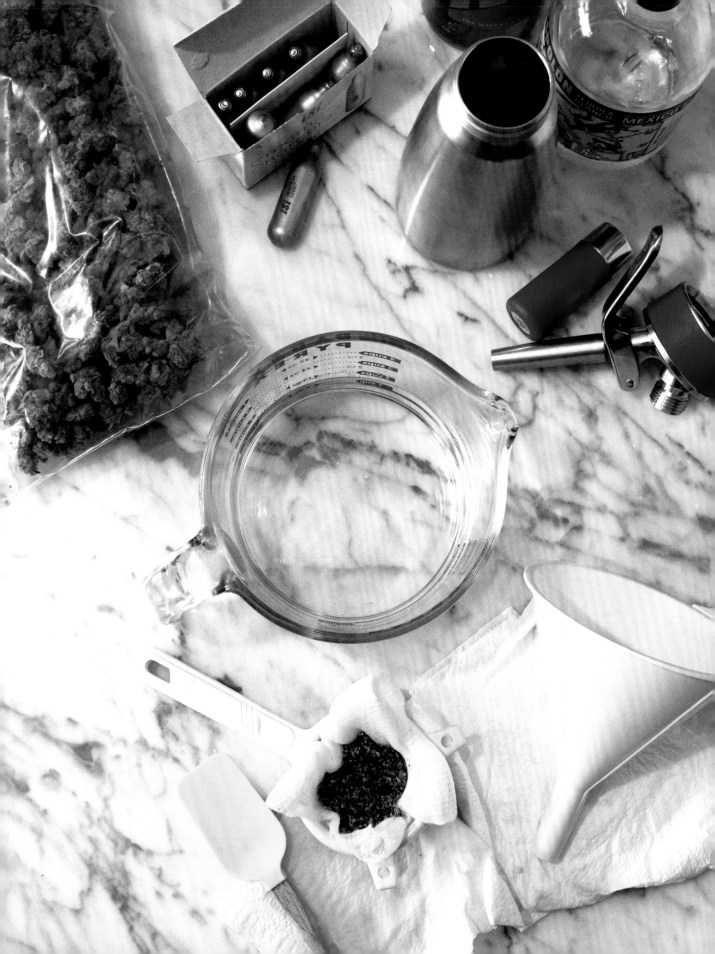

Nitrous Green Dragon

Don Lee

Yield: 2 cups

	THC IN MILLIGRAMS
1 tsp	0.8
1 Tbsp	2.5
¼ cup	10
½ cup	20
¾ cup	30
1 cup	40
2 cups	80

Equipment

0.5-liter heat-tolerant whipped cream dispenser

Nitrous-oxide charger

Two 16-ounce canning jars with lids

Stockpot

Kitchen towel

Silicone oven mitt or jar tongs

Mesh strainer

Cheesecloth

3 grams ground cannabis flower

2 cups mezcal

By using a nitrous oxide–powered whipped-cream dispenser to "force infuse" cannabinoids into liquor, legendary New York City bartender Don Lee created a gorgeous, transparent emerald booze that actually tastes really good. This once-revolutionary method quickly became the favored way to create basic ingredients for cannabinated cocktails, sparking a rush of interest from high-minded mixologists far and wide. There are other ways to infuse cannabis into alcohol that don't require a whipped-cream dispenser, but if you're serious about creating weed cocktails, this is the way to do it! It works for infusing any alcohol, from mezcal (called for here) to gin, whiskey, brandy, tequila, and more.

Put the cannabis material and mezcal in the canister of the whipped-cream dispenser. Screw on the dispenser head and charge with the nitrous-oxide charger according to the manufacturer's instructions. Let the canister sit for 5 minutes.

Vent out the pressurized gas. Stir the liquid and then let it sit for a minute, until the gas boils off. (At this point, the liquor will be imbued with cannabis flavor but won't have developed much THC potency. The next step decarboxylates the weed liquor, making it

continued

potent as well as cannabis-flavored.) Pour the mezcal-weed mixture into a canning jar and seal the top loosely.

Stand the jar upright in the stockpot and add water until it is level with the alcohol. Place the stockpot, uncovered, over medium heat and bring to a simmer. Let simmer for 1 hour, checking the water every now and again and adding more as needed to maintain the original level.

After 1 hour, lay the kitchen towel on a heatproof work surface. Using the oven mitt, remove the jar from the water, set it on the towel, and let cool until it can be handled.

Line the strainer with the cheesecloth and strain the mezcal into the second jar, squeezing the solids at the very end to extract all of the alcohol. Compost or discard the plant matter.

Store in a cool, dark place for up to 6 months. Use sparingly, the combined effects of mezcal and cannabis are intense; the recommended serving size is just 1½ ounces in any cocktail.

INFUSING ALCOHOL

If you want to make cannabis cocktails, you can infuse weed into spirits and use the cannabinated liquors to create mind-bending concoctions. Most traditional recipes involve little more than steeping together alcohol and cannabis in a cool, dark place for several months. But crafty stoners recently figured out improvements to increase potency and speed production time by adding heat and/or pressure.

Traditionally, highly concentrated alcohol-based tinctures were used as folk remedies. These same tinctures can be diluted in drinks, replacing infused liquors, to create cannabis cocktails.

Using Everclear, a popular brand of high-proof grain alcohol, to create a tincture will yield the highest potency product. Unfortunately, it tastes awful and burns when dropped under the tongue. Many commercially available tinctures trade out grain alcohol in favor of grape spirits distilled from wine, which are 85 percent proof alcohol by volume compared to 95 percent for Everclear.

Pro Tip: We made our infusions into alcohol with dried and cured flower that had not been decarboxylated because we wanted to preserve the cannabis flavor, but you could use decarb'ed flower to increase the psychoactivity of these drinks if desired.

Vanessa Says: Alcohol and cannabis are a tricky combo; we've infused gins and served wine on the show. Balance is key, but I think wine and cannabis can be a classic pairing. The terpenes, the terroir—they complement each other well. Also, there's an anecdotal theory that it is best to smoke then drink, rather than the other way around.

Everclear Cannabis Tincture

MUNCHIES Test Kitchen

Yield: ½ cup

	THC IN MILLIGRAMS
1 tsp	14.3
1 Tbsp	43
¼ cup	172
½ cup	344.3

Equipment

8-inch round tempered-glass pie plate

Saucepan large enough to fit pie plate on top snugly

Mesh strainer

Cheesecloth

Liquid measuring cup

7 grams cannabis flower, ground and decarboxylated (see page 55)

One 375-ml bottle Everclear

This basic recipe for a cannabis tincture can be used not only for making cocktails but also for the pepperoni recipe from chef Justin Severino on page 239. Don't go drinking this; the flavor is harsh and it's very potent, but Everclear does its best work in this recipe.

In the pie plate, combine the cannabis flower and Everclear.

Half fill the saucepan with water, set over high heat, and bring to a boil. Set the pie plate over the saucepan, turn the heat to medium, and allow the alcohol to evaporate slowly until the liquid is reduced by half, 45 to 60 minutes. Remove from the heat and let cool.

Line the strainer with the cheesecloth and strain the alcohol into the measuring cup, squeezing the solids at the very end to extract all of the tincture. Compost or discard the plant matter.

Use right away, or transfer to a small clean jar, cap tightly, and store in a cool, dark place for up to 6 months.

Pro Tip: Infusing flammable alcohol over a gas flame is dangerous; so be careful. If you can, use an electric burner; or at the very least, make sure you have plenty of ventilation.

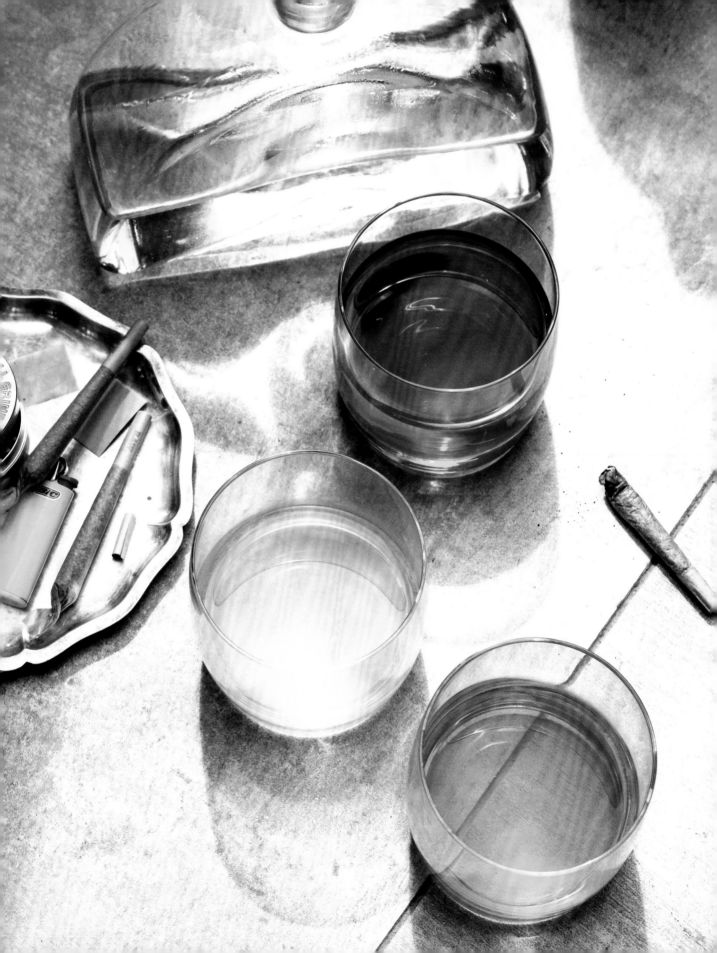

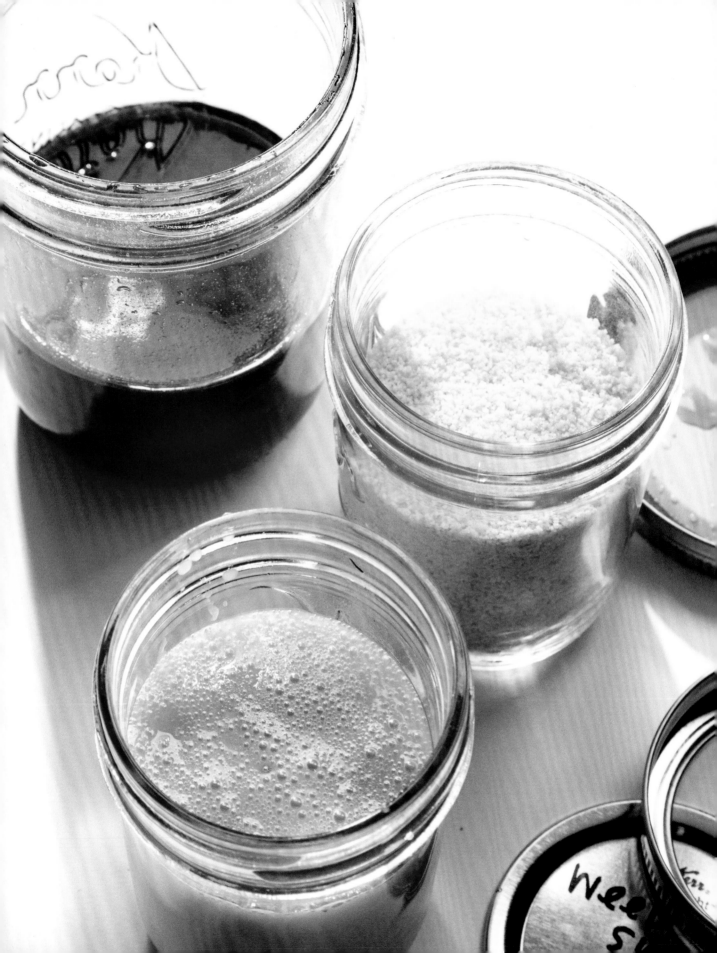

Glycerin Cannabis Tincture

MUNCHIES Test Kitchen

Yield: 1 cup

	THC IN MILLIGRAMS
1 tsp	13
1 Tbsp	39
¼ cup	156
½ cup	312
1 cup	624

Equipment

16-ounce canning jar

Stockpot

Kitchen towel

Silicone oven mitt or jar tongs

Mesh strainer

Cheesecloth

Liquid measuring cup

1 cup organic food-grade glycerin

7 grams cannabis flower, ground and decarboxylated (see page 55)

This basic recipe for a glycerin-based cannabis tincture can be used to infuse cocktails, sauces, and desserts; Forbidden Fruit flowers turned this one (pictured opposite, top left) deep purple. If you find yourself adding just small amounts of it to drinks or the like, store in a dark-colored glass bottle with an eye dropper for ease of dosing.

Pour the glycerin into the canning jar. Add the cannabis flower and stir to mix. Seal the jar tightly.

Stand the jar upright in the stockpot and add water until it is level with the top of the jar. Place the stockpot, uncovered, over high heat and bring to a low boil. Lower the heat and simmer for 2 hours, checking the water every now and again and adding more as needed to maintain the original level. After the first hour, "burp" the jar by unsealing the lid to release any pressure buildup and then recap it.

After 2 hours, lay the kitchen towel on a heatproof work surface. Using the oven mitt, remove the jar from the water, set it on the towel, and let cool completely. Line the strainer with the cheesecloth and strain the tincture into the measuring cup, squeezing any solids at the very end to extract all of the tincture. Compost or discard the plant matter.

Use right away, or transfer to a clean small jar and store in a cool, dark place for up to 6 months.

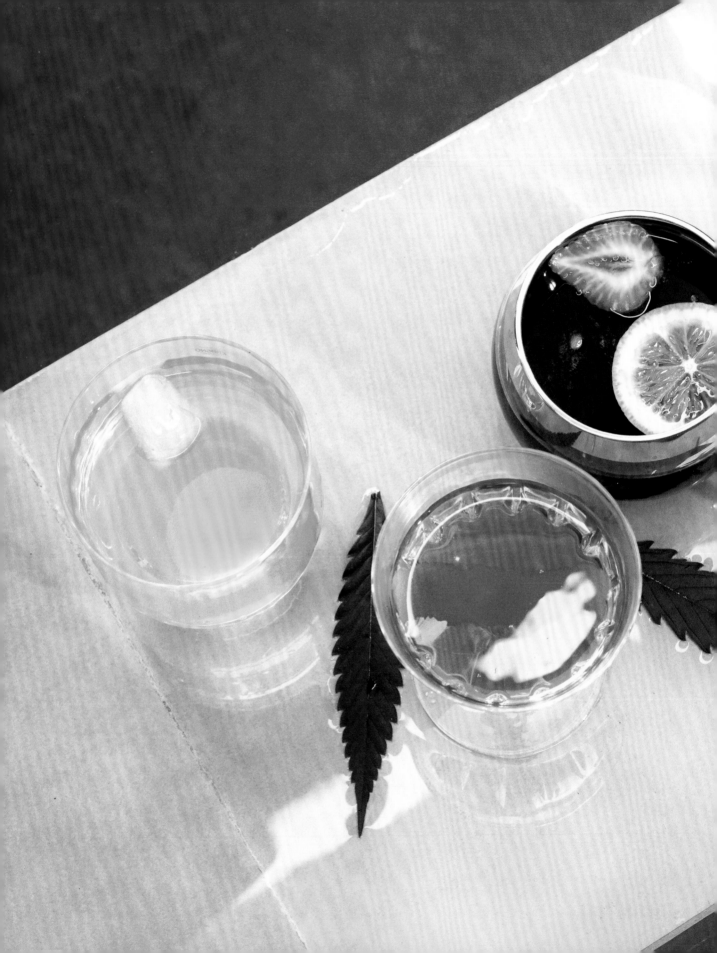

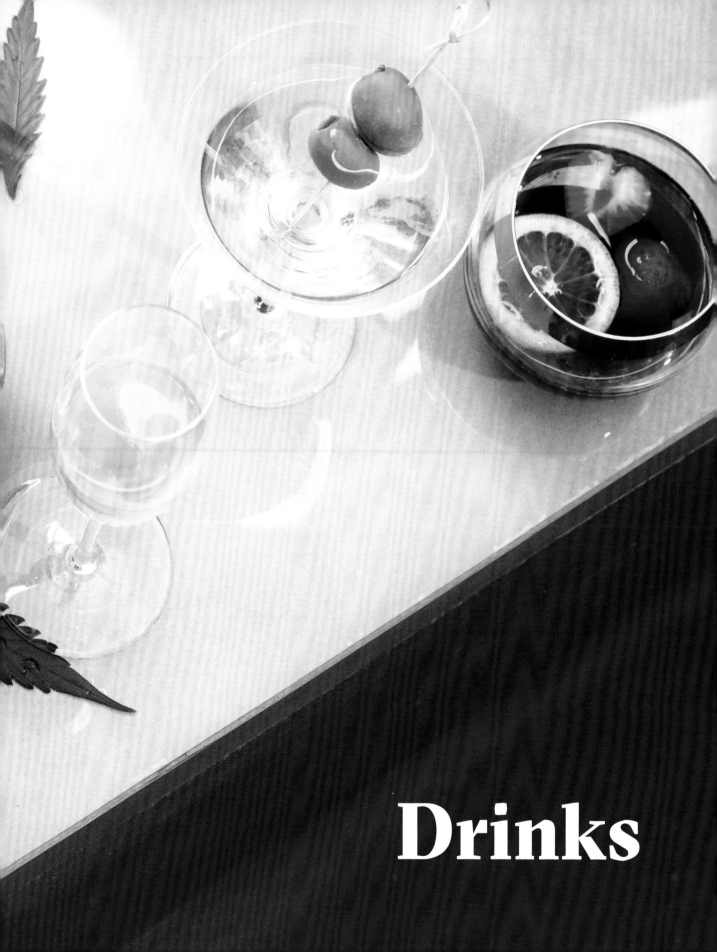

Drinks

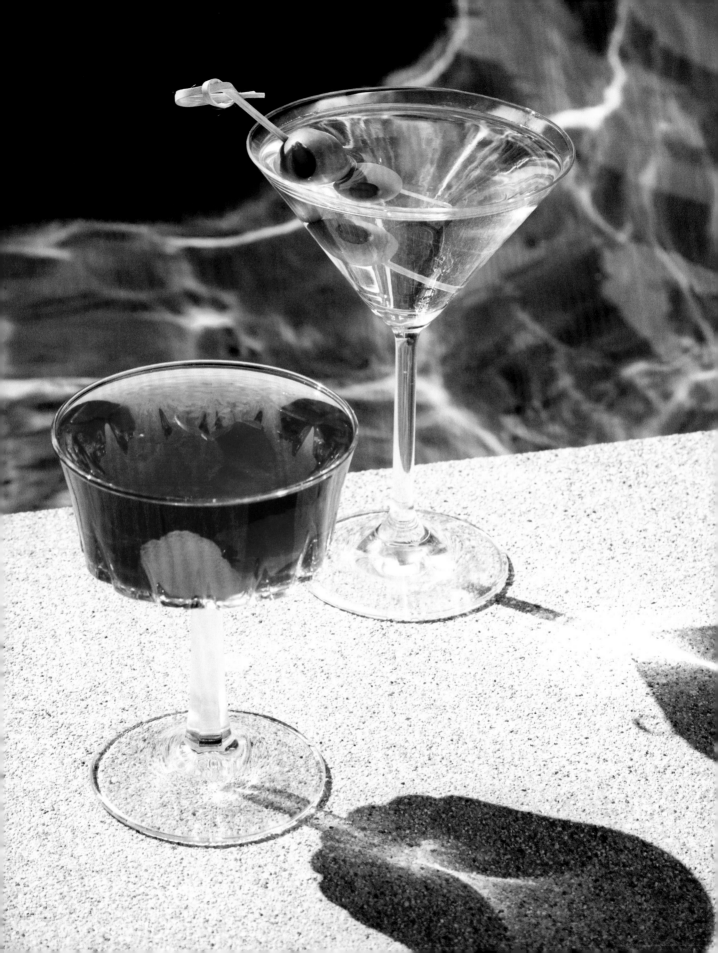

THC
6 mg per cocktail

Manhattan

MUNCHIES Test Kitchen

Yield: 1 cocktail

1 ounce weed-infused whiskey (see Nitrous Green Dragon, page 77)

½ ounce sweet vermouth

1 or 2 dashes Angostura bitters

Orange peel twist or Luxardo-brand maraschino cherry for garnish

The herbal undertones of sweet vermouth get another layer of herb with infused whiskey in this mellow version (pictured opposite, left) of a traditional drink, perfect for pairing with a cold night and a glowing fireplace. Infusing your whiskey with a strong citrusy strain like Tangie would make this Manhattan extra-special.

Chill a coupe. Half fill a mixing glass or a cocktail shaker with ice; add the whiskey, vermouth, and bitters; and stir with a bar spoon for 20 to 30 seconds. Strain into the chilled glass and garnish with an orange twist before serving.

THC
5 mg per cocktail

Dirty Martini

MUNCHIES Test Kitchen

Yield: 1 cocktail

1 ounce gin

1 ounce weed-infused gin (see Nitrous Green Dragon, page 77)

¼ ounce dry vermouth

¼ ounce olive juice

Spanish olives for garnish

Martinis are amazing because they're basically a socially sanctioned way to drink an entire glass of gin, by itself, in public. And if you're already going to do that, you may as well add some bud to it, too. A gassy strain such as Sour Diesel or OG Kush, or a pinene-rich weed like Bubba Kush, Trainwreck, or Chemdog would complement the intense savory flavors from the olive juice that make this martini (pictured opposite, right) so dirty.

Chill a martini glass. Half fill a mixing glass or a cocktail shaker with ice; add both gins, the vermouth, and olive juice; and stir with a bar spoon for 20 to 30 seconds. Strain into the chilled glass and garnish with the olives before serving.

White Negroni

Daniel Nelson
Yield: 1 cocktail

1 ounce weed-infused gin
(see Nitrous Green Dragon,
page 77)

1 ounce Cocchi Americano

1 ounce Herbal-Infused
Vermouth (recipe follows)

Orange peel twist for garnish

Daniel Nelson, partner at The Black Cat on Los Angeles's Sunset Boulevard, is an OG marijuana mixologist and pioneer in the field. He's been making cocktails at weed dinners, both secret and open, for a long time, and was among the first bartenders to openly share his approach to mixing booze and weed. For this crystal-clear riff on a classic Negroni (pictured opposite, right), he uses vermouth infused with both lavender and cannabis (such as Lavender Haze or Amnesia Haze) to amp up the drink's floral and herbal notes. The usual Campari gets replaced with Cocchi Americano, a clear vermouth steeped with botanicals, including bitter cinchona bark and citrus peel.

For the infused vermouth, simmering the lavender releases terpenes into the mix, making for a reliable way to preserve flavors. Source lavender in the fresh-herb section of a well-stocked grocery store. This recipe doesn't add psychoactive THC to the liquor, but it will add weed flavor.

Combine the gin, Cocchi Americano, and vermouth in a mixing glass and stir with a bar spoon. Pour over ice in a rocks glass and garnish with an orange twist before serving.

Herbal-Infused Vermouth

Yield: 1½ cups

One 375-ml bottle dry vermouth

2 tablespoons fresh lavender flowers

1 gram favorite cannabis flower, freshly ground (optional)

In a small saucepan over medium heat, combine the vermouth, lavender, and cannabis flower and bring to a simmer. Let simmer for 3 minutes, then remove from the heat and let cool.

Line a strainer with cheesecloth and strain the cooled vermouth into a measuring cup.

Use right away, or transfer to a bottle, cap tightly, and store in the refrigerator for up to 3 weeks.

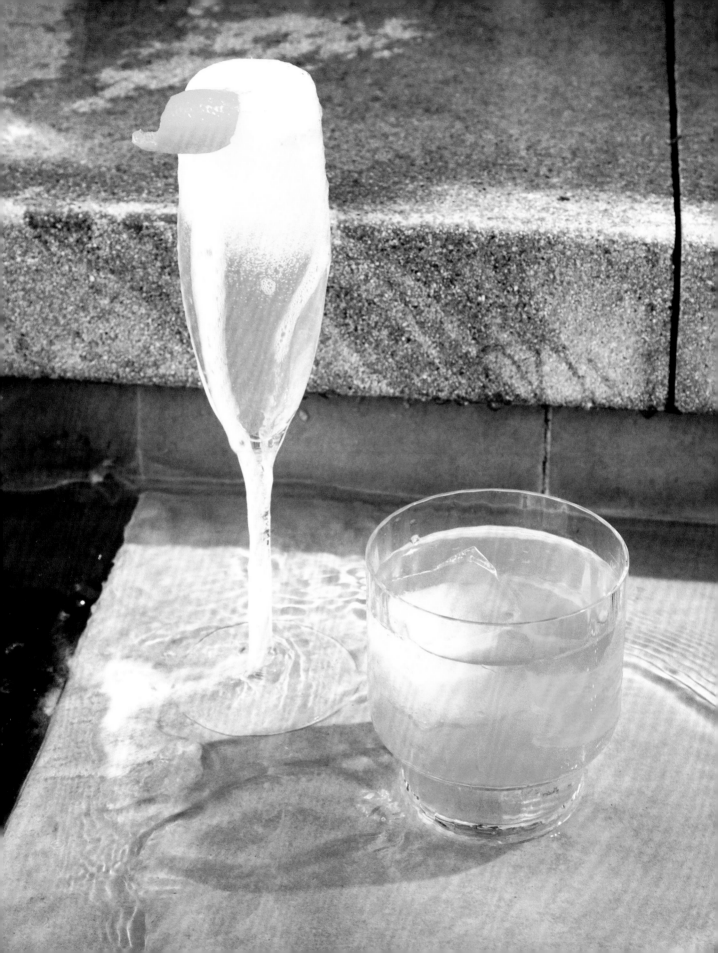

French 75

MUNCHIES Test Kitchen
Yield: 1 cocktail

1 ounce weed-infused gin
(see Nitrous Green Dragon,
page 77)

½ ounce freshly squeezed
lemon juice

2 dashes simple syrup
(recipe follows)

Champagne for topping

Lemon twist for garnish

More like a French 420, amirite? An ultra-chill 5 milligrams of THC make this classic sparkler (pictured on page 89, left) especially celebratory without getting you too stoned. Infusing your gin with a strain high in limonene, like Super Lemon Haze, brings this cocktail to the next level.

Chill a champagne flute. Fill a cocktail shaker with ice; add the gin, lemon juice, and simple syrup; cover; and shake vigorously for 15 to 20 seconds. Strain into the chilled glass, top with Champagne, and garnish with a lemon twist before serving.

Simple Syrup

Yield: 1 cup

1 cup granulated sugar

1 cup water

In a small saucepan over medium-high heat, combine the sugar and water. Cook, stirring occasionally, until the sugar dissolves. Remove from the heat and let cool completely before using.

Store in an airtight container in the refrigerator for up to 3 months.

THC
2.4 mg per serving;
9.44 mg total recipe

Sangria

MUNCHIES Test Kitchen

Yield: 4 servings; 8¾ cups

One 750-ml bottle red wine

2 cups apple juice

¼ cup weed-infused brandy
(see Nitrous Green Dragon,
page 77)

¼ cup orange liqueur

2 tablespoons freshly squeezed
lemon juice, plus 2 lemons,
thinly sliced crosswise

5 fresh strawberries, hulled and
thinly sliced

4 small, sticky fresh cannabis
flowers right off a plant

3¼ cups lemon-flavored
sparkling water

We got weed into this sangria (pictured on page 92, top) a couple of different ways. We dropped a few fresh, sticky buds straight off the plant into the wine and let it sit overnight, which got us started with a flavorful (but not psychoactive) base. If you're in this for the psycho-active properties, you'll want to up the ante a little with infused brandy. The higher alcohol content of brandy means it can absorb more THC, packing a significantly higher punch than wine. Use your favorite red wine blend for this; no need to sacrifice an expensive single varietal for sangria. (A few winemakers, like Pax Mahle at Wind Gap Wines, are currently making wine that gets bud folded in during the fermenta-tion process so the end product is both flavored and dosed. But those bottles are hard to come by. That said, if you can get weed wine and want to use it in this, we're definitely not going to stop you. Just be sure you figure in the higher dosage.)

In a large pitcher, combine the wine, apple juice, brandy, orange liqueur, lemon juice, sliced lemons, strawberries, and cannabis flowers and stir well. Cover and refrigerate for at least 4 hours or preferably overnight. Stir in the sparkling water and serve in glasses over ice.

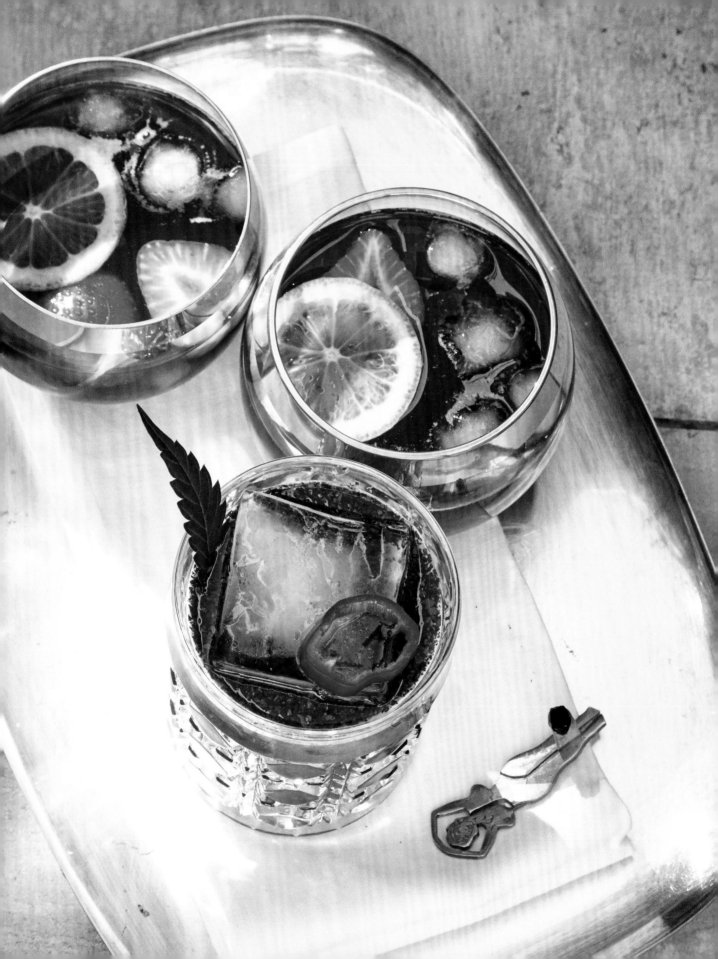

Margarita

Tim Hollingsworth

Yield: 1 cocktail

8 cannabis leaves, each about 2 inches in diameter

1½ ounces weed-infused blanco tequila (see Nitrous Green Dragon, page 77)

¾ ounce freshly squeezed lime juice

¾ ounce grapefruit liqueur (such as Giffard Pamplemousse)

¾ ounce simple syrup (see page 90)

1 pinch kosher salt

2 thin slices fresh bird's-eye or other hot chile

At his restaurant Otium in Los Angeles, Chef Tim Hollingsworth blends peppery nasturtium leaves into a hyper-green cocktail that he rounds out with grapefruit liqueur, hot bird's-eye chile, and infused blanco tequila. But for us, he swapped in cannabis leaves, which, while they're not psychoactive, add a grassy herbal backbone to this refreshing drink (pictured opposite, bottom). If you can't find cannabis or nasturtium in your backyard, you can use a little arugula.

In a blender, combine seven of the cannabis leaves, the tequila, lime juice, grapefruit liqueur, simple syrup, salt, and a chile slice and blend on high speed for 10 seconds.

Fill a cocktail shaker with ice, pour in the blended mixture, cover, and shake for 10 seconds, until the shaker ices over slightly.

Pour the contents over ice in a rocks glass and then garnish with the remaining cannabis leaf and chile slice before serving.

THC

7.5 mg per cocktail

With cannabis flower:
About 17.5 mg

Apple Bong

Devon Tarby

Yield: 1 cocktail

1 large Red Delicious or
other red apple

½ lemon

1½ ounces weed-infused
mezcal (see Nitrous Green
Dragon, page 77)

1 ounce apple juice

½ ounce freshly squeezed
lemon juice

½ ounce simple syrup
(see page 90)

1 drop XJ-13 terpenes (optional)

0.5 gram cannabis flower (such
as Jack Herer or XJ-13) for
smoking

Of course you know what an apple bong is. You're human after all, and you probably also went to high school. But cocktail-hero Devon Tarby of L.A.'s Honeycut and The Normandie Club wants you to take apple carving from a furtive dorm-room pursuit to a much more soigné experience.

Here, an apple (the favorite of every teacher's pet) gets hollowed out and filled with a cocktail built around smoky weed-infused mezcal—Devon recommends Bruxo's Espadín—that gets even smokier as you hit the bong. The smokiness of the mezcal pairs naturally with cannabis flavors like XJ-13 or Jack Herer, a particularly good choice for infusing the liquor as well as smoking through the apple pipe. Amp up the flavors by adding a drop of XJ-13 terpenes to the cocktail if you can get your hands on them. Sip a little, smoke a little, sip a little more. Bong water never tasted so good.

Carefully cut off the top (stem end) of the apple and rub the exposed flesh with the lemon half. Cover the top and put aside. Next, carve out the apple flesh (eat or use for juice), creating a small bowl with ¼-inch-thick sides for holding the drink. Rub the inside of the apple with the lemon half, cover the apple bowl, and put aside.

Fill a cocktail shaker with ice; add the mezcal, apple juice, lemon juice, simple syrup, and terpenes (if using); cover; and shake vigorously for 15 to 20 seconds. Strain into the apple bowl (the whole cocktail might not fit, so have a glass on the side in case there is extra).

Take a straight stiff straw and push it through one side of the reserved apple top, then remove any flesh from the straw. Next, make a small reservoir on the apple top. The hole should be big enough to allow smoke to pull through, but not so large that your weed will fall into the cocktail. Place the apple top back on the apple, put the cannabis flower in the reservoir, and take a sip of the cocktail. Once there is enough headroom inside the apple (about ¼ inch), light the bowl. Enjoy your high and the smoky flavor of the rest of the cocktail.

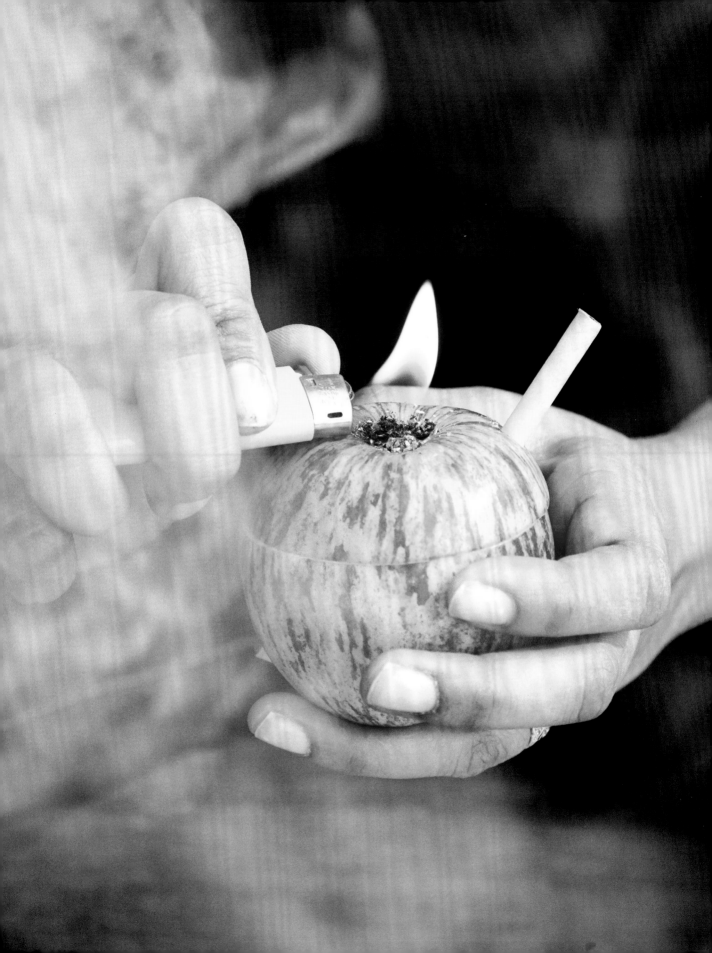

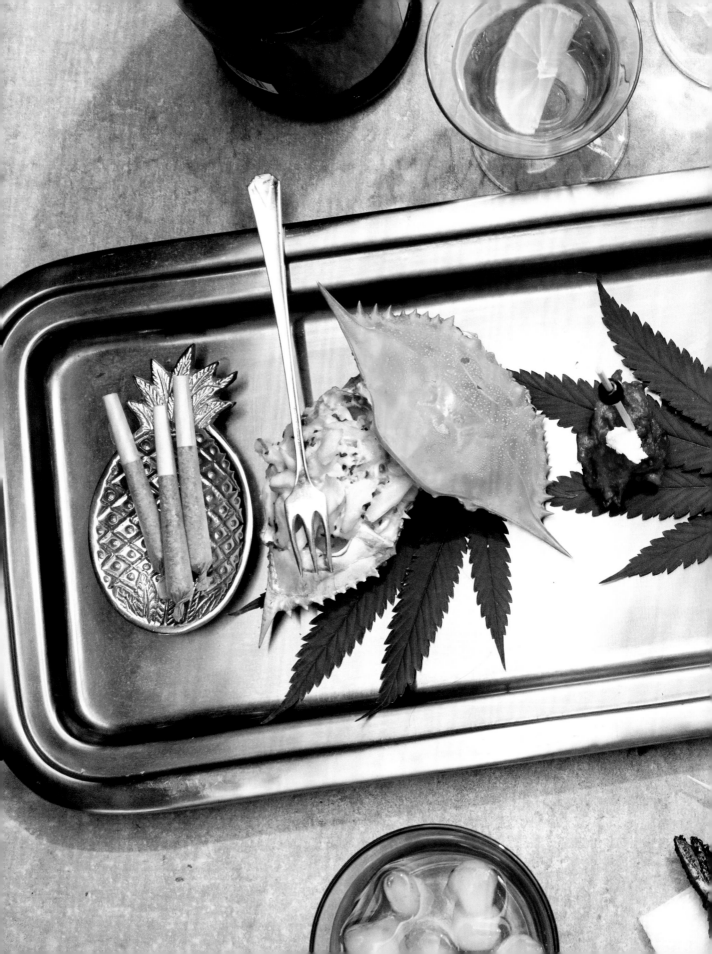

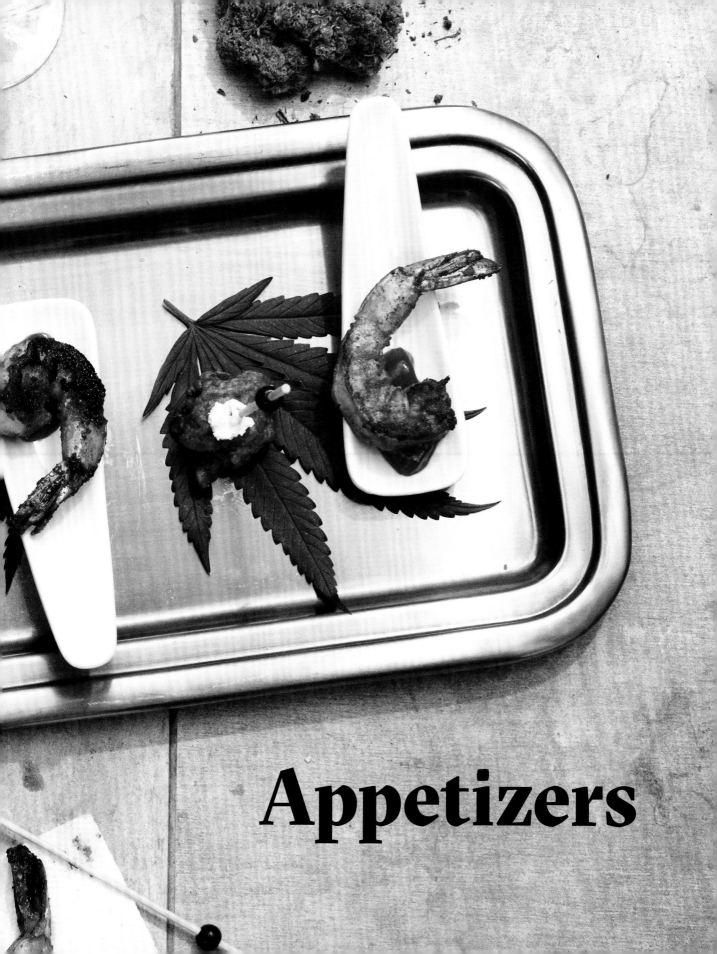

Appetizers

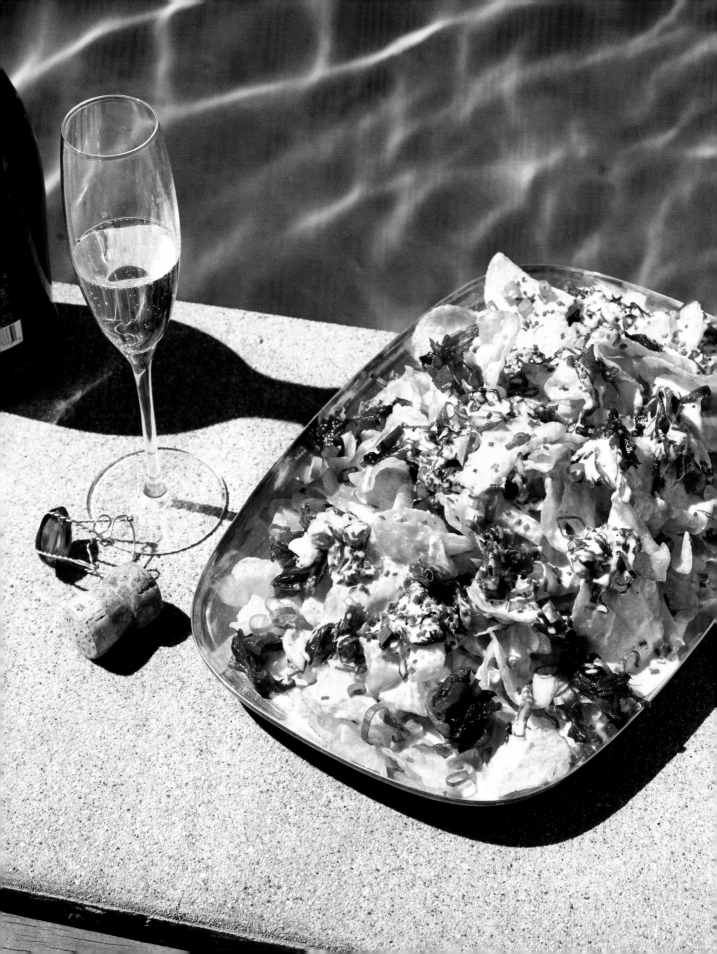

THC
4.2 mg per serving;
16.7 mg total recipe

With weed-infused cream:
12.6 mg per serving;
50.2 total recipe

Sour Cream and Onion Nachos

MUNCHIES Test Kitchen

Yield: 4 servings

3 tablespoons unsalted butter

1 tablespoon flower-infused butter (see page 68)

1½ pounds yellow onions, thinly sliced

1¾ cups plus 3 tablespoons heavy cream

1 tablespoon weed-infused cream (see page 72; optional)

½ cup sour cream

1 teaspoon garlic powder

1 teaspoon onion powder

Kosher salt

One 8-ounce bag kettle-style potato chips

3 green onions, white and tender green parts, thinly sliced

1 bunch chives, finely chopped

You can take chips and dip from our cold, dead hands. But still, you know what's better than chips and dip? Potato-chip nachos layered with caramelized onions and drizzled with warm, weed-laced sour cream sauce. You can either caramelize your onions in a little bit of flower-infused butter, or you can add weed-infused cream to the sour cream sauce—or both. Live large.

In a skillet over medium heat, melt both the butters. Add the yellow onions and cook, stirring occasionally, for about 1 hour, until deeply golden and caramelized. Remove from the heat and keep warm.

In a saucepan over medium heat, bring the heavy cream to a simmer. (If using the weed-infused cream, add it now.) Cook for about 15 minutes, until thickened and reduced by almost half. Stir in the sour cream, garlic powder, and onion powder and season with salt, mixing the cream sauce well. Remove from the heat.

Spread the chips on a serving platter and top with the caramelized onions. Drizzle with the cream sauce and sprinkle with the green onions and chives. Serve warm.

Vanessa Says: Add the infused cream for an extra THC boost. Using a variety rich in caryophyllene, such as OG Kush, will add a peppery note to the dish.

THC
4.7 mg per pakora;
281.5 mg total recipe

Red Beet Pakoras

Fatima Ali

Yield: 60 pakoras

Goat Cheese Sauce

½ cup crumbled fresh
goat cheese

2 tablespoons plain
Greek yogurt

1 teaspoon flower-infused
olive oil (see page 64)

Juice of 1 orange

Kosher salt and freshly ground
black pepper

Pakoras

2 tablespoons coriander seeds

1 tablespoon ground cumin

1 teaspoon chili powder

0.5 gram raw kief

3 red beets, peeled and
coarsely grated

3 cups chickpea flour, plus
more as needed

Kosher salt

1 large cannabis fan leaf,
finely chopped

1½ cups soda water

Canola oil for frying

Fatima Ali runs Van Pakistan, a killer food truck that feeds Pakistani-inspired dishes, such as buttermilk fried chicken biryani, to hungry crowds at Brooklyn's Smorgasburg. When she came through the *Bong Appétit* kitchen, she blew everyone away with these gorgeous beet fritters, which will completely change your perspective on the generally yawn-worthy combo of beets and goat cheese.

To make the goat cheese sauce: In a small bowl, combine the goat cheese, yogurt, infused olive oil, and orange juice and mix well. Season with salt and pepper, cover, and refrigerate until ready to use.

To make the pakoras: With a mortar and pestle, grind together the coriander seeds, cumin, chili powder, and kief until fine. Transfer to a large bowl. Add the beets, chickpea flour, 1 tablespoon salt, cannabis leaf, and soda water and stir to form a loose batter. As the batter sits, the beets will release liquid, so add more chickpea flour as needed to maintain a good consistency.

Pour the canola oil to a depth of 3 inches in a large, wide, heavy saucepan and heat to 375°F on a deep-frying (candy) thermometer. Line a large baking sheet with paper towels. Heat the oven to 200°F.

Working in batches to avoid crowding, drop heaping teaspoons of the batter into the hot oil and fry, turning the fritters as needed to cook and color evenly, until lightly golden and crispy, about 4 minutes. Using a slotted spoon, transfer the pakoras to the prepared baking sheet and keep warm in the oven. Repeat until all of the batter has been fried.

Season the pakoras with salt, then transfer to a serving plate and serve hot with the goat cheese sauce.

Pro Tip: When deep-frying something that contains raw kief, the heat of the fryer can activate more of the THCA, converting it to THC. You're frying these fritters for only 4 minutes, so it's unlikely that much more decarboxylation will occur.

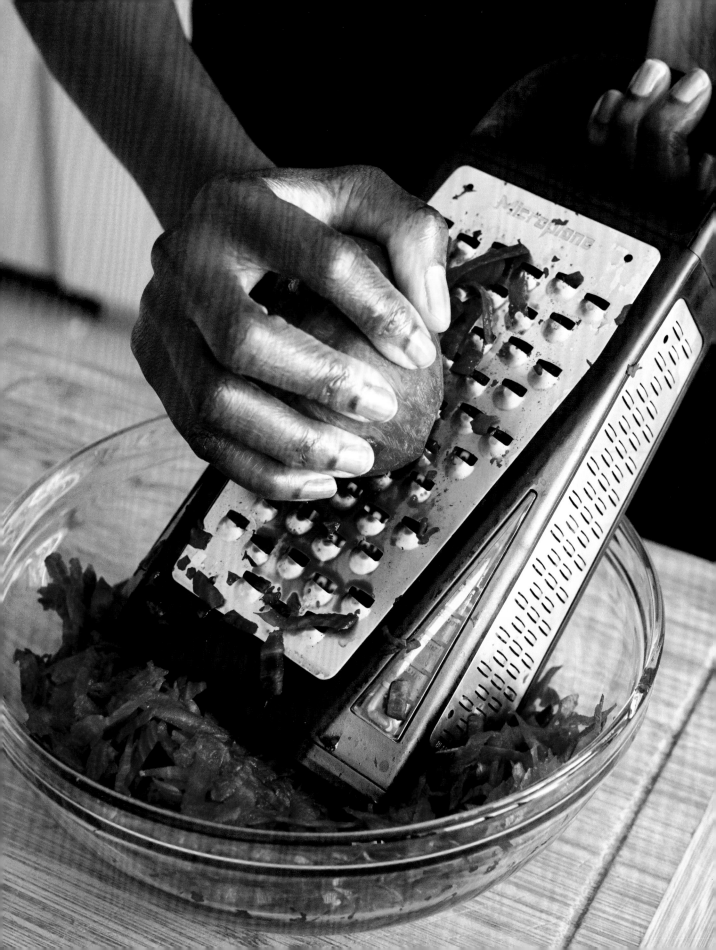

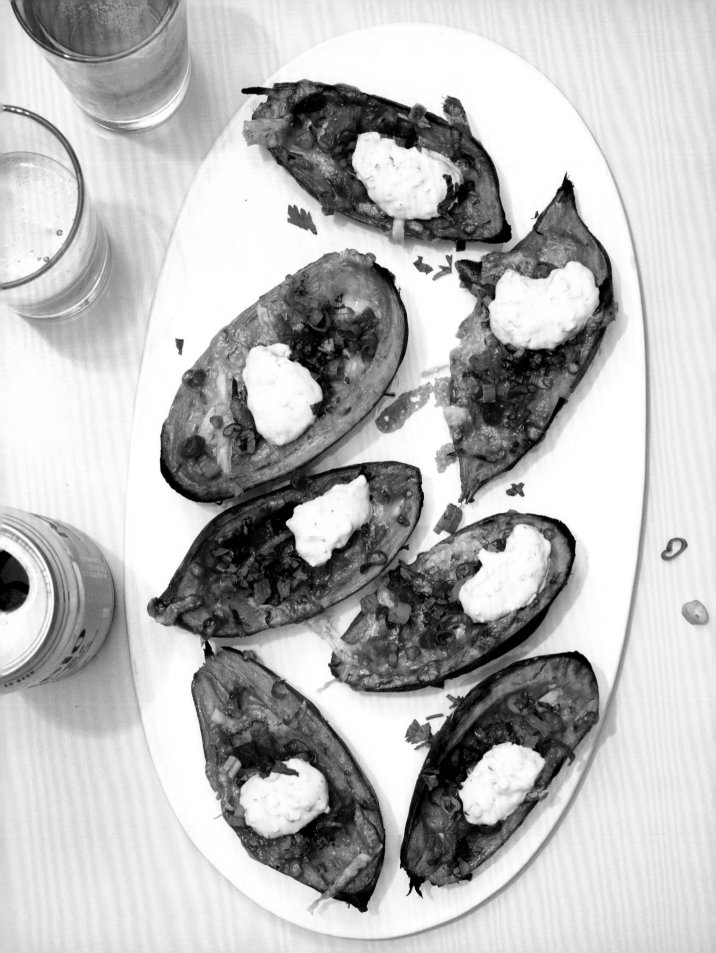

THC
3.5 mg per potato skin;
28.6 mg total recipe

Sweet Potato Skins with Pancetta and Chipotle Crema

Melissa D'Elia

Yield: 8 potato skins

Weed-Infused Pancetta Fat

1 pound pancetta, in a single piece, cut into ¼-inch cubes

1 gram cannabis trim, ground and decarboxylated (see page 55)

½ cup crème fraîche

2 tablespoons minced fresh basil

2 tablespoons minced fresh cilantro

2 tablespoons minced fresh mint

1 tablespoon minced chipotle chile in adobo sauce

2 green onions, white and tender green parts, thinly sliced

4 sweet potatoes, scrubbed

2 cups grated Gruyère, raclette, or smoked Gouda cheese

Melissa D'Elia is a private chef with years of cannabis cooking experience (it's a hard job, but someone has to do it). One of the big takeaways she's gleaned over time is that if you're making something people are going to want to eat a lot of, you need to keep the dose low so folks don't accidentally end up too blazed to function. These potato skins fit the bill: they're ultra-low dose but ridiculously addictive. If this all feels like a lot to do at once (infusing the fat takes about 3 hours), you can infuse the pancetta fat and bake the potatoes ahead of time. Use any leftover infused pancetta fat for frying eggs on chill weekend mornings.

To make the weed-infused pancetta fat: Line a plate with paper towels.

In a large skillet over medium heat, cook the pancetta, stirring occasionally, until crispy and the fat has rendered, about 6 minutes. Using a slotted spoon, transfer the pancetta to the prepared plate and set aside. Pour the remaining fat into a 12-ounce canning jar, stir in the trim, and seal tightly.

Stand the jar upright in a stockpot and add water until it is level with the top of the jar. Place the stockpot, uncovered, over high heat and bring to a low boil. Let boil for 2 hours, checking the water every now and again and adding more as needed to maintain the original level. After the first hour, "burp" the jar by unsealing the lid to release any pressure buildup and then recap it.

After 2 hours, lay a kitchen towel on a heatproof work surface. Using an oven mitt, remove the jar from the water, set it on the towel, and let cool until it can be handled. Then, while the fat is still liquid, line a strainer with cheesecloth and strain the fat into a measuring cup,

continued

squeezing any solids at the very end to extract all of the fat. Compost or discard the plant matter. Set aside.

In the bowl of a food processor, combine the crème fraîche; 1 tablespoon each of the basil, cilantro, and mint; the chile; and 2 tablespoons of the green onions. With the motor running, drizzle in 2 tablespoons of the infused pancetta fat, processing until well mixed. Transfer the crema to a airtight container and refrigerate until ready to use.

Heat the oven to 450°F.

Wrap the sweet potatoes individually in aluminum foil and place on a baking sheet. Bake for about 1 hour, until tender when pierced with a fork. Remove from the oven and let cool slightly. Leave the oven on.

Halve the warm sweet potatoes lengthwise. Scoop out the flesh from each half, leaving walls about ½ inch thick (save the removed flesh for another use). Place the potatoes, skin-side down, on the baking sheet and rub each one with 1 teaspoon of the infused pancetta fat, then sprinkle with the cheese and the cooked pancetta, dividing it evenly.

Bake the skins for about 20 minutes, until golden and crispy. Transfer to a serving platter and top each skin with 2 tablespoons of the crema. Sprinkle with the remaining 1 tablespoon each basil, cilantro, and mint and the remaining green onions, dividing them evenly. Serve immediately.

THC
0.9 mg per spring roll;
110 mg total recipe

Fried Spring Rolls

Christine Hà

Yield: 25 spring rolls

Spring Rolls

**1 ounce dried wood ear
mushrooms**

**2 ounces bean thread noodles,
hydrated according to package
instructions**

**½ carrot, peeled and coarsely
chopped**

**¼ yellow onion, coarsely
chopped**

**2 ounces backfin crabmeat,
picked over for shell and
cartilage fragments**

1 garlic clove, thinly sliced

½ shallot, thinly sliced

¼ pound ground turkey

1½ tablespoons fish sauce

0.5 gram raw kief

1 large egg, lightly beaten

**Twenty-five 8½-inch round
rice-paper wrappers**

Dipping Sauce

1 garlic clove, grated

**1 fresh red chile, seeded
(if desired) and minced**

Juice of 1 lime

½ cup water

¼ cup fish sauce

**¼ cup plus 2 tablespoons
granulated sugar**

Canola oil for frying

Lettuce leaves for serving

These Vietnamese-style spring rolls pack a riot of flavors into tight little packages. Writer and television host Christine Hà, who goes by "The Blind Cook," has an incredible palate, which she puts to tremendous use building layers of flavor into everything she makes. On the show, Hà crumbled Diablo OG flower directly into the filling for these rolls, but we're going with raw kief here for a more controlled dose. Raw kief isn't nearly as potent as decarboxylated kief, so there's a lot of acidic THCA remaining in this ingredient. The quick but intense heat of the deep fryer may activate more THC, making the potency of these rolls variable.

Although you will be able to find some of the Asian-specific ingredients at any well-stocked supermarket, it is probably best to stop by your local Asian grocery store and pick up wood ear mushrooms, bean thread noodles, fish sauce, and rice paper wrappers all at once.

To make the spring rolls: Bring a small pot of water to a boil over high heat. Remove from the heat, add the mushrooms, and let sit for 10 minutes; then drain, discarding the water.

In the bowl of a food processor, combine the mushrooms, noodles, carrot, and onion and pulse until finely chopped. Transfer to a medium bowl.

Add the crab, garlic, and shallot to the food processor and pulse until smooth. Transfer the crab mixture to the bowl with the mushroom mixture, then add the turkey, fish sauce, kief, and egg and stir to mix well. Cover the filling and refrigerate for 1 hour.

Have ready a wide shallow bowl or pie plate of room-temperature water and a large platter or tray.

Submerge a rice-paper wrapper in the water just until softened and pliable, about 20 seconds, then transfer it to a work surface. (Do not leave it in the water too long or it will soften too much and tear.) Place 2 tablespoons of the filling near the closest edge of the

continued

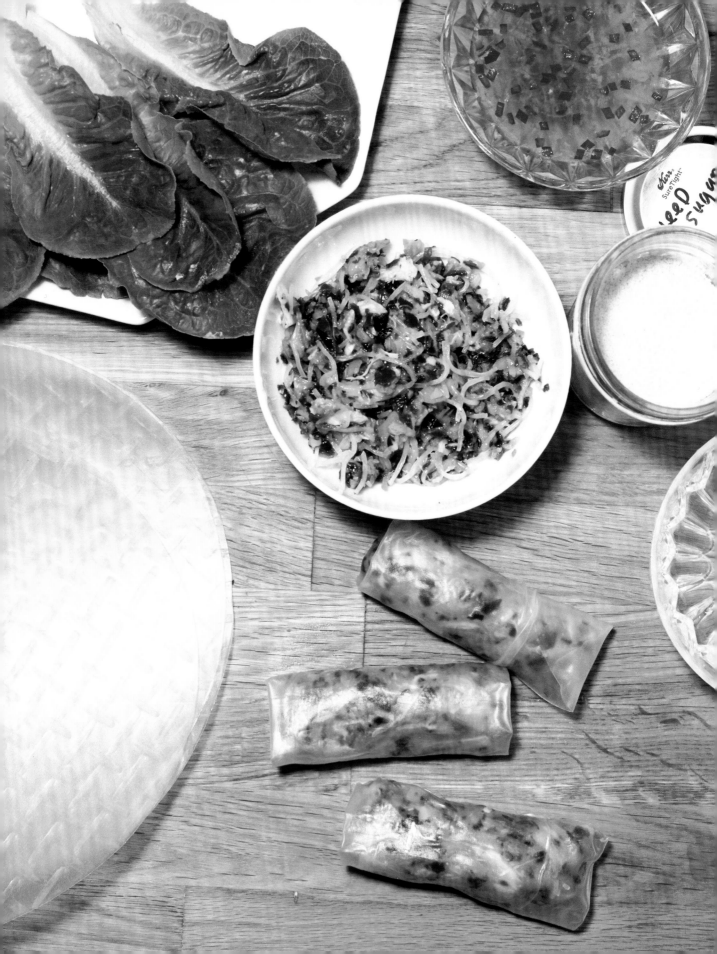

Fried Spring Rolls, *continued*

wrapper. Roll the wrapper edge closest to you up and over the filling. Fold in the left and right sides of the wrapper, continue rolling away from you, tucking tightly as you go, until you reach the top edge, then press to seal the seam securely. Repeat with the remaining rice-paper wrappers and filling, setting the rolls aside, seam-side down, on the platter as they are ready.

To make the dipping sauce: In a small canning or other jar with a tight-fitting lid, combine the garlic, chile, and lime juice. In a small bowl, whisk together the water, fish sauce, and sugar until the sugar has dissolved. Add the fish sauce mixture to the jar, cover tightly, and shake to combine. Use right away, or store in the refrigerator for up to 2 weeks.

Pour the canola oil to a depth of 2 inches in a large, wide, heavy saucepan and heat to 350°F on a deep-frying (candy) thermometer. Set a large wire rack on a baking sheet. Heat the oven to 200°F.

Working in batches to avoid crowding, add the rolls to the hot oil and fry, turning the rolls as needed to cook and color evenly, until golden and crispy, about 8 minutes. Using tongs, transfer the rolls to the wire rack and keep warm in the oven.

Serve the rolls warm with lettuce leaves and dipping sauce. Invite everyone to wrap a warm roll in a lettuce leaf before dipping.

Vanessa Says: Crumbling Diablo OG adds a textural element to the dish as well as spicy flavors. Crumble some into your spring roll filling for an extra kick.

THC

0.5 mg per wonton;
11.3 mg total recipe

With ¼ cup dipping sauce:
4.7 mg; 18.9 mg total recipe

Dipping Sauce

½ cup red pepper flakes

1½ teaspoons kosher salt

½ teaspoon granulated sugar

3 garlic cloves, grated

¾ cup plus 3 tablespoons
canola oil

1 tablespoon flower-infused
canola oil (see page 64)

Wontons

½ pound ground pork

½ cup finely chopped fresh
garlic chives

2 tablespoons black vinegar

2 tablespoons soy sauce

1 tablespoon peeled and grated
fresh ginger

3 garlic cloves, grated

0.25 gram raw kief

Twenty 3½-inch square
wonton wrappers

Pork Wontons

Nom Wah Tea Parlor
Yield: 20 wontons and 1 cup sauce

Nom Wah Tea Parlor, a much-loved dim sum spot, has been a fixture in New York's Chinatown since 1920. Although plenty has changed in the world since then, Nom Wah's dumpling game remains entirely on point. While weed-infused chile-garlic dipping sauce isn't something you'll find on the menu, it's a killer addition to these spicy, savory wontons. If you're feeling bold, you can shake a little raw kief into the ground pork filling to make these dumplings a little more potent, or you can dose just the dipping sauce to keep things chill. You can usually find wonton wrappers in a well-stocked supermarket, but will likely need to visit an Asian market for the black vinegar (rice based and inky black) and garlic chives (long, green, and flat, with a faint garlic aroma).

To make the dipping sauce: In a small heatproof bowl, combine the red pepper flakes, salt, sugar, and garlic. In a small saucepan over medium heat, combine both oils and warm to 240°F on a deep-frying (candy) or laser thermometer. Pour the hot oil into the bowl and whisk to mix well. Let cool for 1 hour, then use right away, or cover and refrigerate for up to 1 month.

To make the wontons: In a large bowl, combine the pork, chives, vinegar, soy sauce, ginger, garlic, and kief and mix well.

Line a baking sheet with parchment paper and have a small bowl of water nearby.

Line up about ten of the wonton wrappers on your work surface. Place about 2 teaspoons of the pork mixture in the center of a wrapper and, using a fingertip dipped in the water, lightly dampen the outside edge of the wrapper. Fold the wrapper in half to form a triangle, taking care to press out any air pockets and pressing the edges to seal well. Now fold the two bottom corners of the triangle together, overlapping them slightly, and seal with a dab of water. Place the finished wonton on the prepared baking sheet. Repeat with the remaining wrappers and filling. (If you like, you can freeze the wontons at this point. Slip the baking sheet in the freezer, and when the wontons are frozen solid, transfer them to a ziplock freezer bag and freeze for up to 2 months.

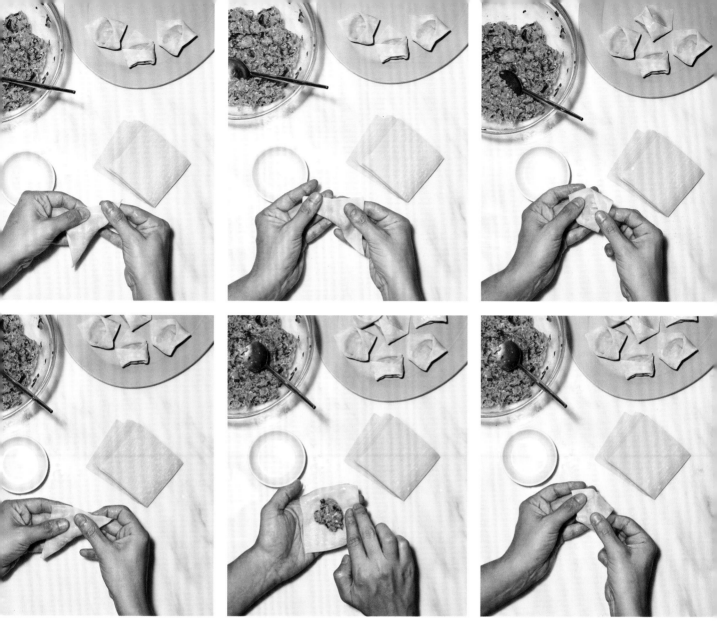

They can be cooked directly from the freezer, adding 1 minute to the cooking time.)

Bring a pot of water to a boil. Add the wontons and cook for about 2½ minutes. They are ready when they float to the surface. (If you want to make sure the filling is cooked through, scoop out a dumpling and check.) Using a wire skimmer, lift them from the pot, shaking off any excess water, and transfer them to a platter. Serve warm with the dipping sauce.

THC
32.8 mg per serving;
130.8 mg total recipe

With Pot Pepperoni:
35 mg per serving;
139.6 mg total recipe

French Bread Pizza

MUNCHIES Test Kitchen

Yield: 4 servings

2 tablespoons flower-infused butter (see page 68)

1 tablespoon unsalted butter

1 tablespoon olive oil

2 garlic cloves, minced

1 yellow onion, thinly sliced

One 28-ounce can whole peeled tomatoes, crushed by hand

Kosher salt and freshly ground black pepper

1 large loaf French bread, halved horizontally

1 pound mozzarella cheese, shredded

1 cup Homemade Ricotta Cheese (page 233)

1 cup thinly sliced Pot Pepperoni (page 239; optional)

Fresh basil or cannabis fan leaves, thinly sliced, for garnish

Red pepper flakes or grated Parmesan cheese for garnish

This is what after-school snacks always hoped to grow up to be. If you're going for total DIY cred, make the ricotta cheese *and* pepperoni; if you're just trying to get high, the chunk of cannabis butter in the tomato sauce will take care of that nicely. (And no, you don't have to use either; or French bread, for that matter. This also makes a killer pizza bagel, pizza ciabatta, or pizza whatever-you-have-in-the-house.)

In a saucepan over medium-high heat, warm both butters with the olive oil. Add the garlic and onion and cook, stirring occasionally, until soft, about 5 minutes. Add the tomatoes and cook, stirring occasionally, until the sauce is thick, 15 to 20 minutes. Season with salt and pepper.

Remove from the heat and let cool slightly. Transfer to a blender and process until smooth.

Heat the broiler.

Place the bread halves, cut-side up, on a baking sheet. Spread about 1 cup sauce on each half and top with mozzarella, ricotta, and pepperoni (if using), dividing them evenly. Slide the baking sheet under the broiler and broil until the cheese is melted and golden and the pepperoni is crispy, about 4 minutes.

Remove from the oven, let cool slightly, and then garnish with basil and red pepper flakes. Cut each bread half in half again and serve.

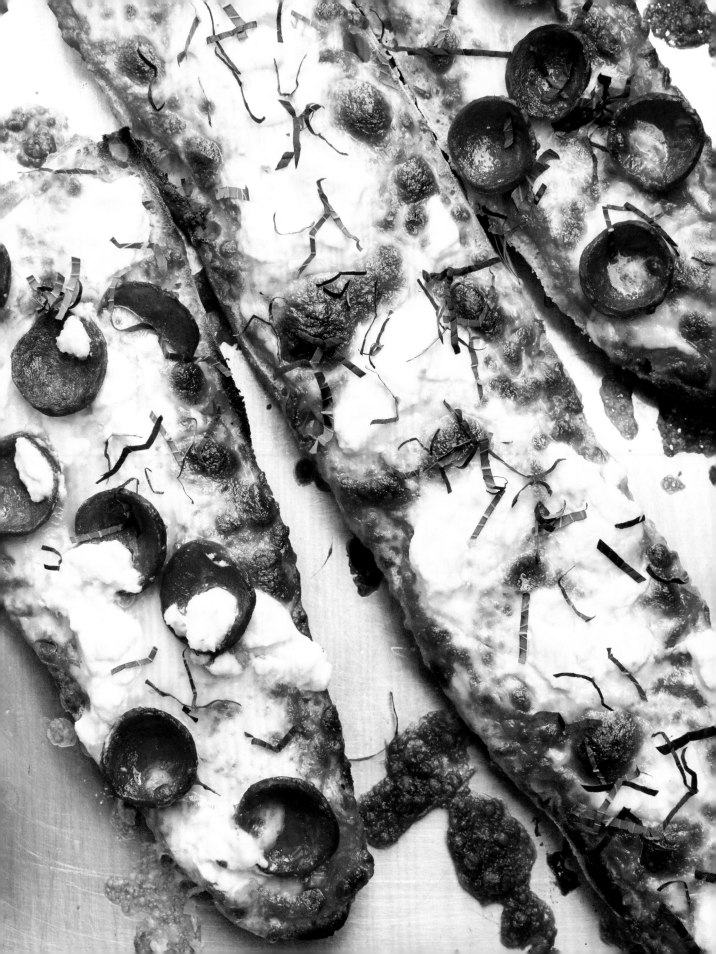

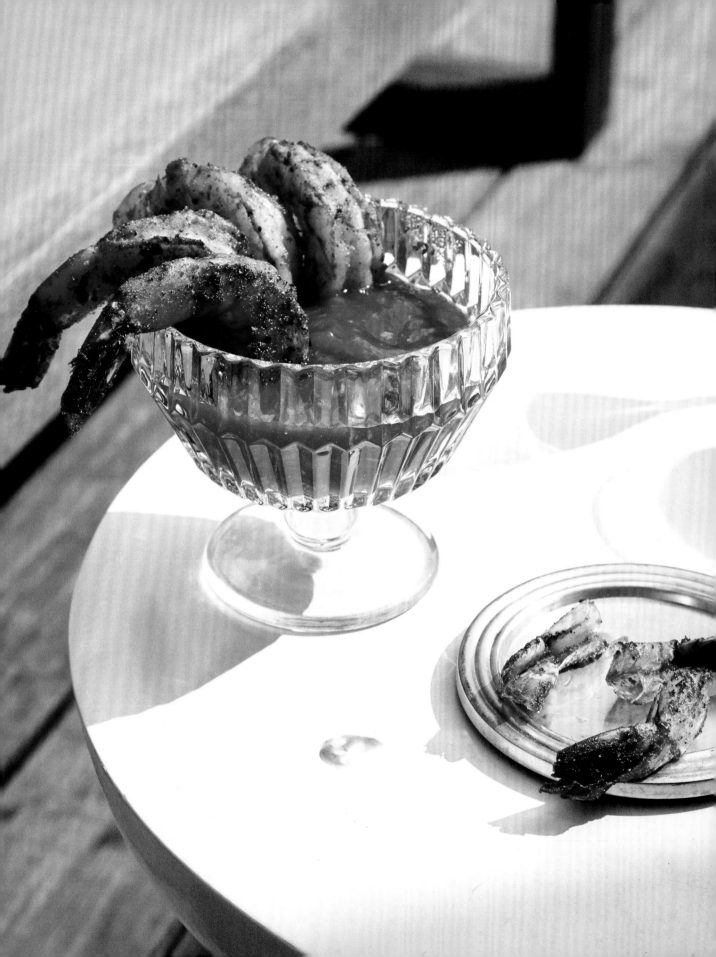

THC

2.6 mg per serving;
10.4 mg total recipe

With kief: 8.6 mg per serving,
44.5 mg total recipe

Blackened Shrimp Cocktail

Courtney McBroom

Yield: 4 servings (3 shrimp per serving) and ½ cup cocktail sauce (2 Tbsp per serving)

Courtney McBroom is a proud Texas native who you absolutely cannot expect to serve you a boring-ass poached shrimp cocktail. Her version blackens the shrimp with a spice blend containing three types of pepper, garlic powder, and onion powder, plus a gram of kief that keeps everybody happy.

Serve them up as old-school as your heart desires! Put the cocktail sauce in the bottom of a martini glass and fan the shrimp out on the rim, with a lemon wedge in the mix for good measure. And, for the love of God, if you happen to have decorative pot leaves on hand, use as many as humanly possible (for flair).

To make the cocktail sauce: In a bowl, combine the ketchup, lemon juice, horseradish, Worcestershire, and infused olive oil and stir to mix well. Cover and refrigerate until ready to use.

To cook the shrimp: In a small bowl, combine the black, white, and cayenne peppers; onion and garlic powders; salt; and kief (if using) and mix well.

Rinse the shrimp and pat dry with paper towels. One at a time, dredge each shrimp in the spice mixture, coating evenly. Be generous, as the more coverage you get, the more flavor you get!

In a large cast-iron or other heavy skillet over medium heat, warm the olive oil until hot and shimmering. Add the shrimp in a single layer and cook them, without disturbing, until the underside is nicely darkened, 1½ to 2 minutes. Flip the shrimp and cook on the second side for 1½ to 2 minutes longer. The shrimp should be opaque throughout. They may burn a bit, and that's okay. You want blackened shrimp, not nicely browned shrimp.

Transfer the shrimp to a plate and serve immediately with the cocktail sauce for dipping. Or, if you prefer to serve them in the classic shrimp-cocktail style, let them cool, then chill, uncovered, in the fridge for at least 30 minutes or up to 1 hour before serving.

Cocktail Sauce

¼ cup ketchup

2 tablespoons freshly squeezed lemon juice

2 teaspoons grated fresh horseradish

1 teaspoon Worcestershire sauce

1 tablespoon flower-infused olive oil (see page 64)

Shrimp

2 teaspoons freshly ground black pepper

2 teaspoons freshly ground white pepper

2 teaspoons cayenne pepper

2 teaspoons onion powder

2 teaspoons garlic powder

2 teaspoons kosher salt

1 gram raw kief (optional)

12 large shrimp, peeled and deveined

2 tablespoons olive oil

Vanessa Says: When choosing a variety of kief, opt for a bright citrus aroma. Sour Diesel or a Super Lemon Haze will work well with the cocktail sauce.

THC
11.7 mg per serving,
93.6 mg total recipe

Coconut Crab Gratin

MUNCHIES Test Kitchen

Yield: 8 servings

1 cup weed-infused coconut milk (see page 71)

2 teaspoons cornstarch

1 pound jumbo lump crabmeat, picked over for shell and cartilage fragments

2 tablespoons minced red onion

1 tablespoon minced fresh cilantro

½ teaspoon coconut sugar or granulated sugar

Grated zest and juice of 1 lime, plus lime wedges for serving

Kosher salt and freshly ground black pepper

Toast points for serving

Cilantro and lime lighten up this delicate, sweet crab starter that's bound with infused coconut milk. If you have your pick of strains for infusing the coconut milk, select something on the citrusy side, like Super Lemon Haze or Tangie. Serving this gratin in natural crab shells is optional but baller. If crab shells are hard to come by, a small baking dish works fine, too.

Heat the broiler.

In a small saucepan, whisk together the coconut milk and cornstarch, then place over medium heat and cook, stirring, until the mixture thickens, 1 to 2 minutes. Remove from the heat and let cool slightly.

Add the crab, onion, cilantro, sugar, lime zest, and lime juice to the coconut milk and stir to mix well, then season with salt and pepper. Divide the crab mixture evenly among the crab shells and arrange the shells on a baking sheet, or spoon the crab mixture into a small broiler-proof baking dish.

Broil until the mixture is golden and bubbling, 3 to 4 minutes. Serve hot with toast points and lime wedges.

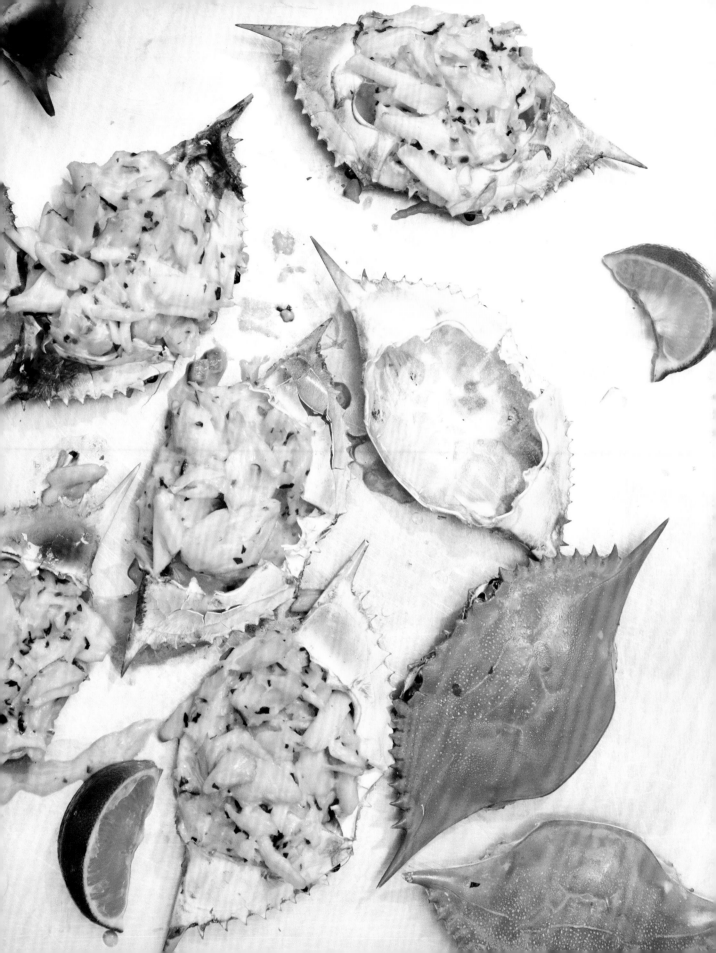

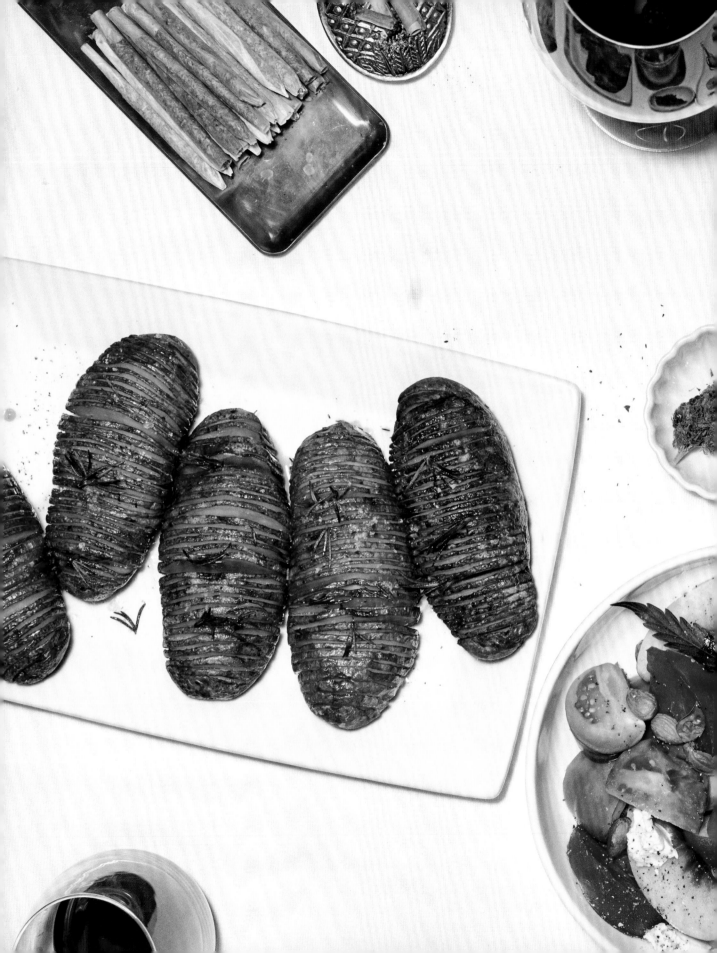

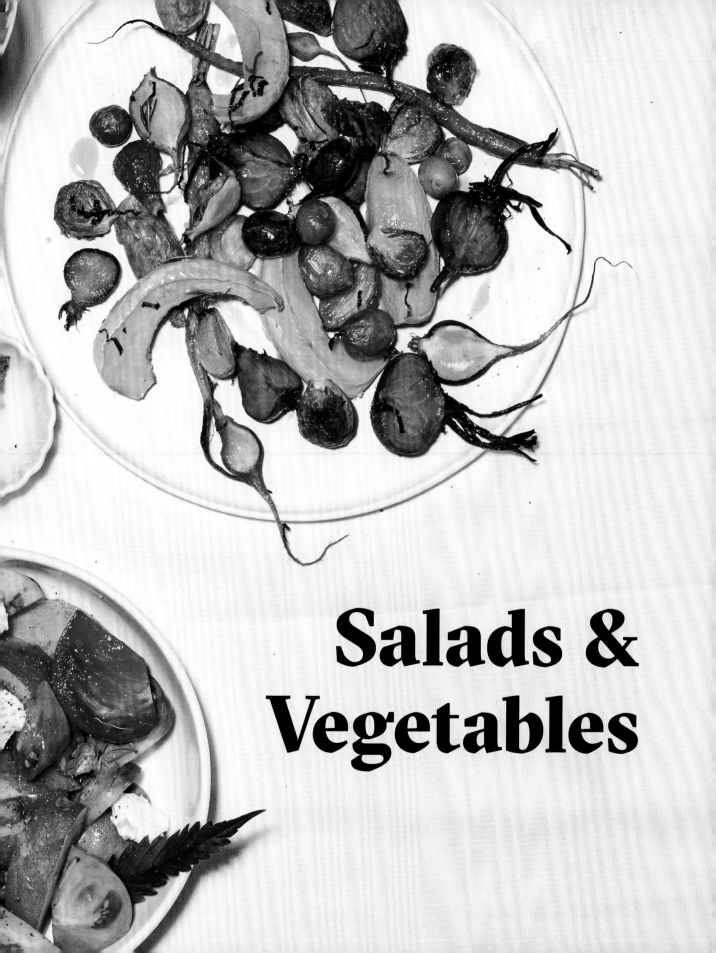

Salads &
Vegetables

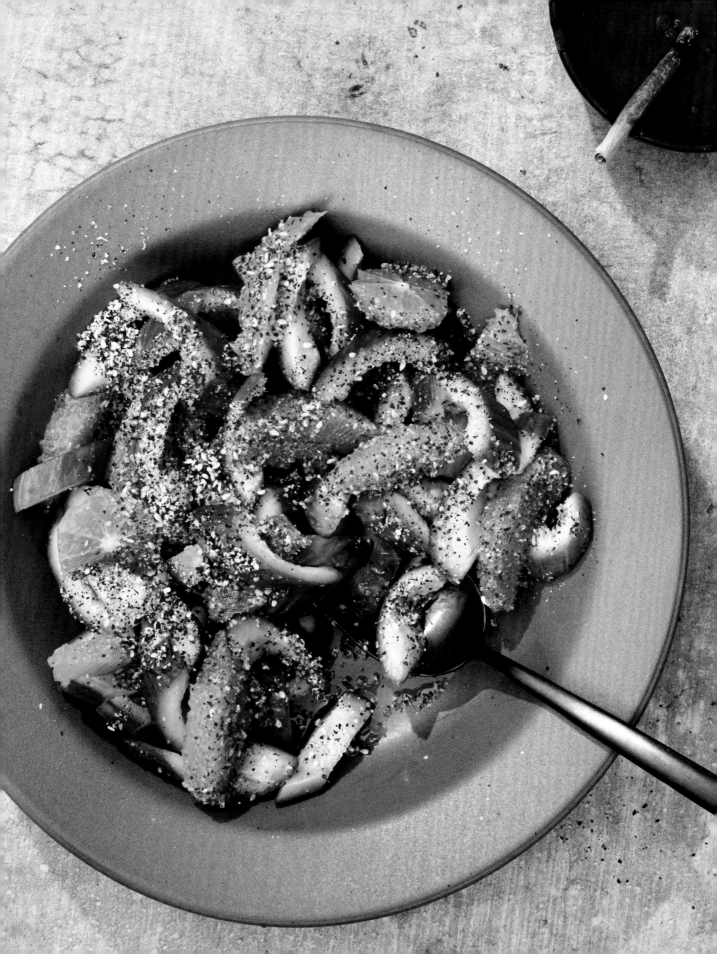

THC
1.7 mg per serving;
6.9 mg total recipe

Cucumber and Citrus Salad

Sarah Hymanson and Sara Kramer/Kismet

Yield: 4 servings

Za'atar

3 tablespoons hemp seeds, lightly ground

3 tablespoons sesame seeds, toasted and lightly ground

2 tablespoons ground sumac

1 teaspoon flower-infused olive oil (see page 64)

8 Persian cucumbers, halved lengthwise, seeded, and sliced crosswise on the diagonal

1 teaspoon flower-infused olive oil (see page 64)

Juice of 2 lemons

Kosher salt

2 mandarin oranges, peeled and segmented

2 blood oranges, peeled and segmented

1 drop Green Crack terpenes (optional)

When Sarah Hymanson and Sara Kramer, usually of Kismet in Los Angeles but also of more cool side projects than we can count, appeared on *Bong Appétit*, they were new to cooking with weed but already total champions with farm-fresh produce, leafy greens, and fresh herbs. Their take on *za'atar*—a popular Middle Eastern seasoning mixture that typically includes thyme and/or oregano, sumac, sesame seeds, and salt—skips the usual herbs in favor of hemp seeds, which won't contribute to a high but do carry plenty of protein. Look for sumac in spice shops or Middle Eastern groceries and hemp seeds in health food or natural foods stores.

To make the za'atar: In a small bowl, stir together the hemp seeds, sesame seeds, sumac, and infused olive oil. The consistency should be such that the mixture is easy to sprinkle. Transfer to an airtight container and store in the refrigerator for up to 3 weeks.

In a medium bowl, toss together the cucumbers, infused olive oil, and lemon juice and season with salt. Add all of the citrus segments and the terpenes (if using) and toss well. Transfer to a serving bowl, sprinkle with za'atar, and serve immediately.

Vanessa Says: To brighten this salad and add some leafy greens, chiffonade some fan leaves to sprinkle on top. Did you know they pack more nutrients than kale?

THC
5.2 mg per serving;
20.8 mg total recipe

With Homemade Ricotta
Cheese: 21.2 mg per serving;
84.8 mg total recipe

Summer Tomato and Stone Fruit Salad

Sam Smith/Tusk

Yield: 4 servings

White Wine and Herb Vinaigrette

2 garlic cloves, minced

3 tablespoons white wine vinegar

1 pinch Maldon sea salt

½ cup loosely packed fresh mint leaves, coarsely chopped

½ cup loosely packed fresh flat-leaf parsley leaves, coarsely chopped

6 tablespoons olive oil

2 tablespoons flower-infused olive oil (see page 64)

1 teaspoon crushed Aleppo pepper

Kosher salt

1 pound mixed heirloom tomatoes, cut into wedges, and cherry tomatoes, halved

1 pound nectarines or peaches, halved, pitted, and cut into wedges

½ cup loosely packed fresh basil leaves

1 small red onion, thinly sliced

⅓ cup almonds, toasted

1 cup Homemade Ricotta Cheese (page 233)

Olive oil for drizzling

Crushed Aleppo pepper for sprinkling

At the vegetable-forward, Israeli-inspired Tusk restaurant in Portland, Oregon, chef Sam Smith makes food that he likes to call "aggressively seasonal." This salad embodies that ethos, to an extent. Yes, it's the perfect dish for the height of summer, but the infused ricotta mutes any aggression you might be harboring. And if you're not feeling ambitious enough to make infused ricotta, buy some good ricotta (from the Italian market, please, not from the grocery store, and nothing with added stabilizers) and swap the regular olive oil in the dressing with additional infused olive oil instead.

To make the white wine and herb vinaigrette: In a small bowl, combine the garlic, vinegar, and Maldon salt and let macerate for 5 to 10 minutes. Toss the mint and parsley with the vinegar mixture, then whisk in both oils and the Aleppo pepper. Season with kosher salt and set aside.

In a large bowl, combine the tomatoes and nectarines and toss to mix. Drizzle with the vinaigrette; sprinkle with the basil, onion, and almonds; and toss to coat evenly. Taste and adjust the seasoning if needed.

Transfer the salad to a plate (any liquid left behind in the bowl is great sopped up with bread). Dot the top of the salad with heaping tablespoons of the ricotta. Drizzle with a little olive oil, sprinkle with Aleppo pepper, and serve immediately.

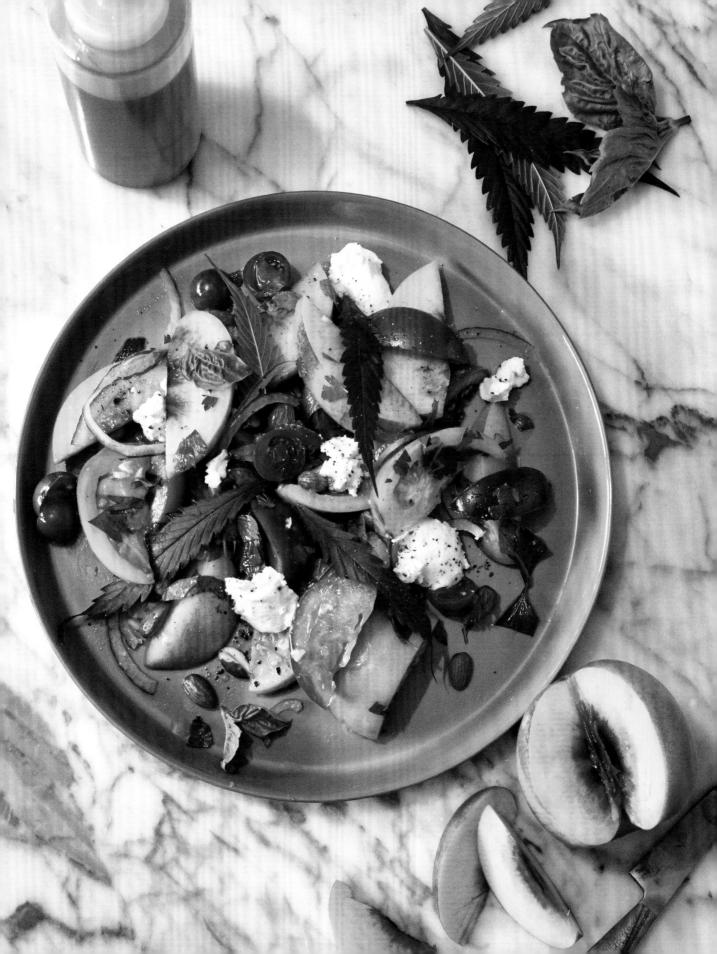

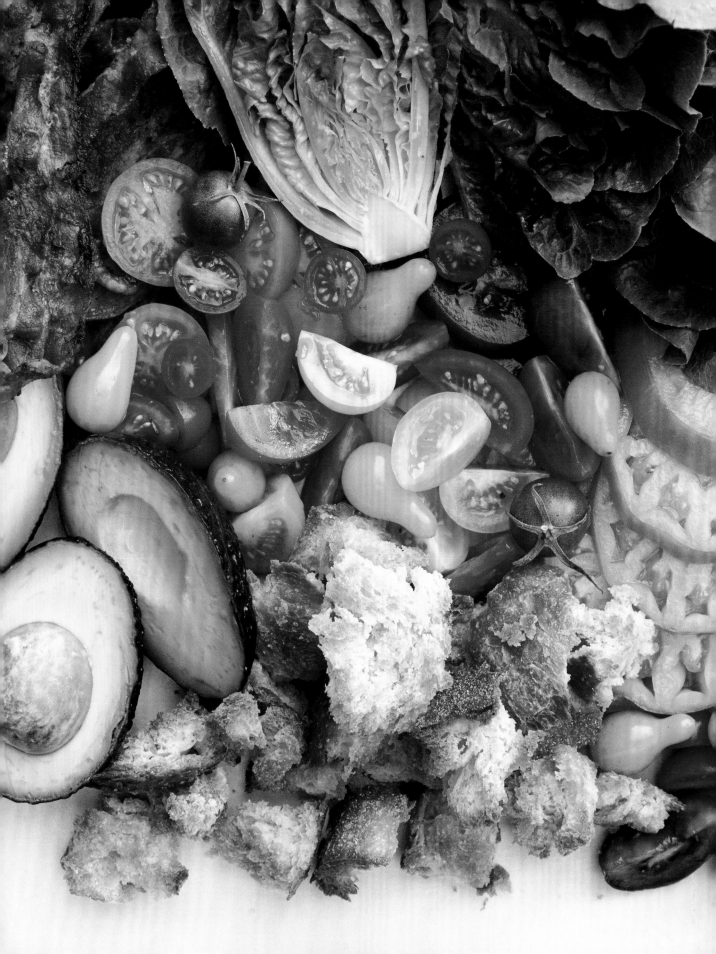

THC
5.2 mg per serving;
31.2 mg total recipe

BLAT Salad

MUNCHIES Test Kitchen

Yield: 6 servings

1 large loaf ciabatta, torn into 1-inch pieces

3 tablespoons olive oil

Kosher salt

1 pound sliced bacon

3 tablespoons flower-infused olive oil (see page 64)

3 tablespoons red wine vinegar

1 pound mixed heirloom tomatoes, thinly sliced, and cherry tomatoes, halved

2 heads romaine lettuce, roughly chopped

2 avocados, halved, peeled, pitted, and diced

Freshly ground black pepper

This is the salad you eat when you're like, "Shit, I should really eat a salad," but you're not willing to go full kale. In other words, this is a salad, but you're still putting bacon, fried bread, and weed in it. Everyone's happy.

Heat the oven to 375°F.

On a large baking sheet, drizzle the bread with the regular olive oil, season with salt, and toss to coat evenly. Spread the bread in an even layer. Bake until golden and crispy, about 10 minutes. Let cool completely.

Meanwhile, line a plate with paper towels.

In a large skillet over medium-high heat, cook as many bacon slices as will fit without crowding, flipping once, until crispy, about 6 minutes on each side. Transfer the bacon to the prepared plate to drain, let cool slightly, then tear into bite-size pieces. Repeat until all the bacon is cooked.

In a large bowl, toss the bread pieces with the infused olive oil and vinegar. Add the bacon, tomatoes, lettuce, and avocados and toss to combine. Season with salt and pepper and serve immediately.

Vanessa Says: If you like bacon as much as I do, infuse the rendered fat with a pinch or two of kief (decarbed for a higher potency) and then toss the bread in a mixture of infused olive oil and the rendered infused bacon fat before toasting in the oven.

THC

12.5 mg per serving;
50 mg total recipe

Creamy Cilantro Kale Salad with Coconut Bacon

Jasmine Shimoda

Yield: 4 servings

1 bunch curly green kale, stems and ribs removed and leaves thinly sliced

½ cup Creamy Cilantro Vinaigrette (facing page)

¼ cup Coconut Bacon (facing page)

1 cup sunflower sprouts

¼ cup sunflower seeds, toasted

20 cherry tomatoes, halved

4 radishes (Purple Ninja or watermelon), peeled and chopped into ¼-inch cubes

4 green onions, white and tender green parts, thinly sliced

3 Persian cucumbers, cut into ¼-inch pieces

1 large avocado, halved, pitted, peeled, and cubed

Kosher salt and freshly ground black pepper

Weed people like to say that cannabis is the new kale. This salad makes it clear that they can share the title. Jasmine Shimoda, of L.A.'s seminal yogi-hangout The Springs, has made more than a few kale salads in her time, and it shows. This one takes everything good about every kale salad you've ever had and synthesizes it into a combination of perfectly tender kale, creamy green goddess-esque dressing (with a wholesome dose of THC), and crunchy smoky coconut "bacon," which might be the only time something that isn't bacon lived up to bacon's good name. Alas, if you don't have a stove-top smoker and a dehydrator, you'll have to skip this inspired addition, but don't worry, the salad won't suffer as a result. The vinaigrette recipe makes more than you need for this salad, but leftovers would be killer smeared on a steak sandwich or used as a dip for crudités if you're fancy.

Put the kale in a large bowl. Drizzle with the vinaigrette, then, using your hands, massage the vinaigrette into the kale for a minute or two, until the kale feels softer. (This step breaks down the tough fibers and releases the natural sweetness of kale.) Add the coconut bacon, sunflower sprouts, sunflower seeds, tomatoes, radishes, green onions, cucumbers, and avocado and toss to mix well. Season with salt and pepper and serve immediately.

THC
25 mg per ¼ cup;
320 mg total recipe

Creamy Cilantro Vinaigrette
Yield: 3 cups

1¼ cups raw cashews, soaked overnight in water to cover

¾ cup plus 2 tablespoons freshly squeezed lime juice

Leaves and tender stems from 1 bunch cilantro, coarsely chopped

1 bunch green onions, white and tender green parts, coarsely chopped

½ jalapeño chile, seeded

Kosher salt

1 cup flower-infused grapeseed oil (see page 64)

Freshly ground black pepper

Drain the cashews, transfer to a blender, and add the lime juice, cilantro, green onions, jalapeño, and 1 tablespoon salt. With the motor running, slowly drizzle in the infused grapeseed oil until emulsified. Season with pepper, then taste and adjust the seasoning with salt. Transfer to an airtight container and store in the refrigerator up to 5 days.

Coconut Bacon
Yield: 2 cups

2 cups unsweetened large coconut flakes

1 tablespoon liquid smoke

½ teaspoon smoked paprika

¼ teaspoon kosher salt

¼ teaspoon freshly ground black pepper

Prepare a stove-top smoker according to the manufacturer's instructions. Add the coconut and smoke for 10 minutes. Then, transfer the coconut to a bowl; add the liquid smoke, paprika, salt, and pepper; and toss to mix well. Spread the seasoned coconut on a dehydrator tray and dehydrate at 115°F overnight, until dry and crispy. Transfer to an airtight container and store at room temperature for up to 2 weeks.

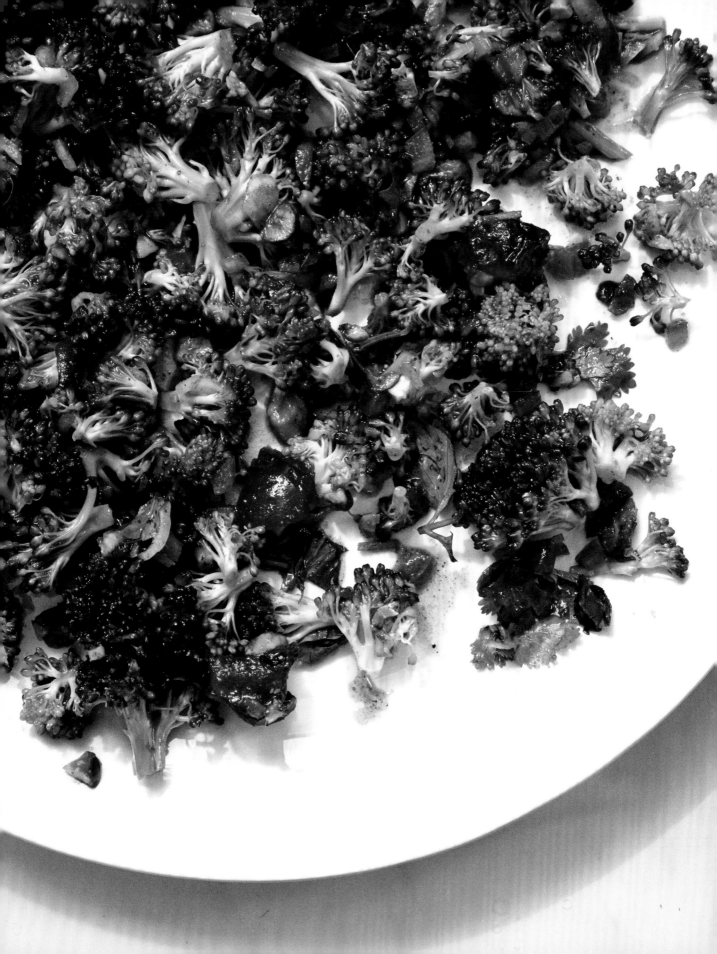

THC
5.2 mg per serving;
20.8 mg total recipe
With whipped infused honey:
7.5 mg per serving;
30 mg total recipe

North African Broccoli Salad

John Clark and Beverly Kim/Parachute
Yield: 4 servings

Ras el Hanout Vinaigrette

2 tablespoons flower-infused olive oil (see page 64)

½ cup plus 2 tablespoons olive oil

2 tablespoons white balsamic vinegar

1 tablespoon ras el hanout

2 small garlic cloves, minced

2 tablespoons freshly squeezed lemon juice

2 tablespoons whipped weed-infused honey (see page 74; optional)

1 large head broccoli, cut into very small florets

¼ cup finely chopped fresh cilantro

¼ cup finely chopped fresh mint

¼ cup pistachios, toasted and finely chopped

10 Medjool dates, pitted and finely chopped

2 small shallots, finely chopped

1 jalapeño chile, seeded (if desired) and finely chopped

Kosher salt and freshly ground black pepper

Vanessa Says: Anytime a recipe calls for herbs, add a few chopped fan leaves. It's a great way to use the whole plant and add a fresh bite to your dish.

This dish from John Clark and Beverly Kim, the husband/wife team behind Chicago's Parachute restaurant, puts the broccoli in broccoli salad—along with dates, *ras el hanout* (a North African spice blend), ground pistachios, cilantro, and mint. It's a series of unexpected flavors that somehow ends up working perfectly together—and it's even better after a day in the fridge.

To make the ras el hanout vinaigrette: In a small saucepan over high heat, combine both oils, the vinegar, ras el hanout, and garlic and bring to a boil. Lower the heat to maintain a steady simmer and cook for 5 minutes. Remove from the heat and strain through a fine-mesh strainer into a small heatproof bowl, discarding the solids. Whisk in the lemon juice and honey (if using). Set aside.

In a large bowl, combine the broccoli, cilantro, mint, pistachios, dates, shallots, and jalapeño and toss to mix. Drizzle with the dressing, season with salt and pepper, and toss to coat evenly. Serve immediately.

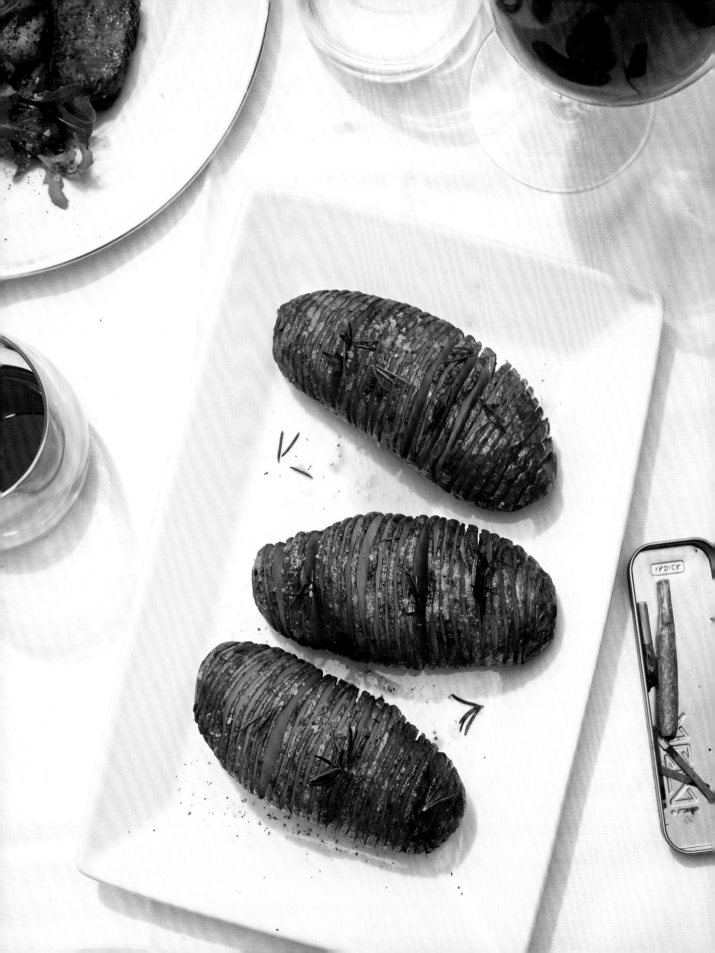

THC
5.2 mg per serving;
41.6 mg total recipe

Hasselback Potatoes

MUNCHIES Test Kitchen

Yield: 8 servings

2 pounds medium russet potatoes, scrubbed

2 rosemary sprigs, broken into many smaller sprigs

¼ cup flower-infused olive oil (see page 64)

¼ cup olive oil

Kosher salt and freshly ground black pepper

These potatoes have the dubious honor of being nearly everyone's favorite carb Instagram post, but they're more than just a pretty face. Slicing potatoes thinly before baking means tons of extra surface area to get crispy-crunchy in the oven—and to absorb all that infused oil.

Heat the oven to 425°F.

Using a sharp knife, cut crosswise slits about ¼ inch apart and about three-fourths through the potato (so the slices remain connected at the bottom) the length of each potato. Place the potatoes on a baking sheet and stuff the slits with the rosemary, dividing it evenly. Drizzle the potatoes evenly with both oils, making sure that the oils reach down into the slits, then season with salt and pepper.

Roast the potatoes until crispy, golden, and cooked through, about 1 hour. Serve immediately.

Roasted Vegetables with Whipped Weed-Infused Honey

MUNCHIES Test Kitchen

Yield: 4 servings

1 pound baby potatoes, halved

¾ pound golden beets, peeled and cut into wedges

⅓ pound baby heirloom carrots, trimmed

½ pound brussels sprouts, trimmed and halved

1 small acorn squash, halved lengthwise, seeded, and thinly sliced crosswise

3 tablespoons olive oil

Rosemary and thyme leaves for sprinkling

Cannabis leaves for sprinkling (optional)

Kosher salt and freshly ground black pepper

¼ cup whipped weed-infused honey (see page 74)

Infused honey fixes a multitude of sins—and plenty of things that aren't sins at all. Here, it works its magic on roasted vegetables, which are a classic for a reason. But they may as well be a classic for a reason that also gets you high.

Heat the oven to 425°F.

On a baking sheet, toss together the potatoes, beets, carrots, brussels sprouts, and squash. Drizzle with the olive oil; sprinkle with the rosemary, thyme, and cannabis (is using); season with salt and pepper; and toss again to coat evenly. Spread the vegetables in a single layer.

Roast the vegetables until golden, crispy, and tender, about 30 minutes. Let cool slightly, transfer to a serving dish, drizzle with the infused honey, and toss gently. Serve immediately.

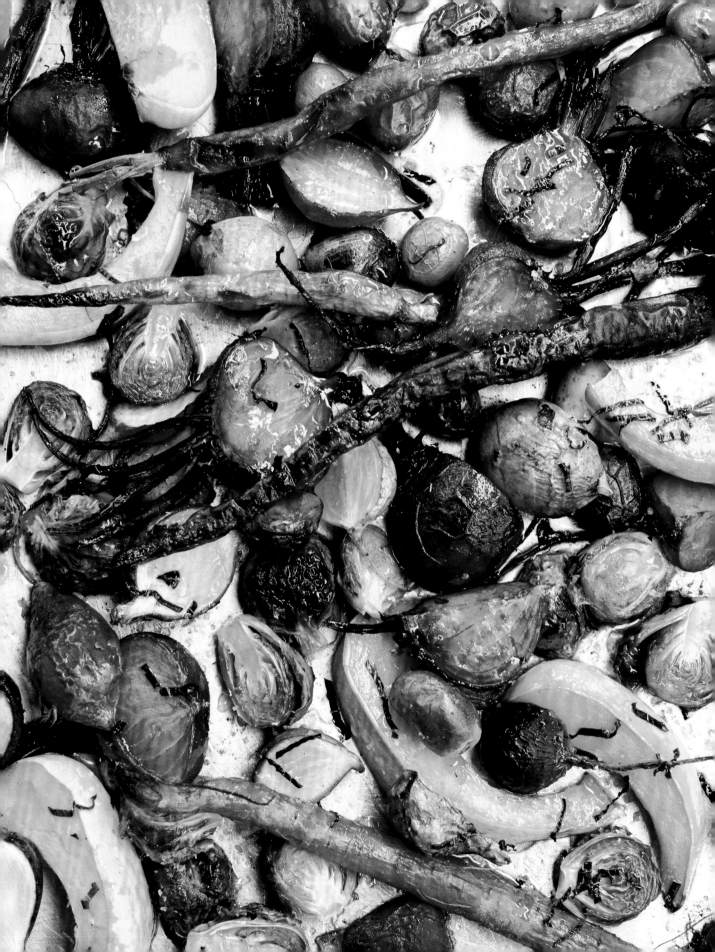

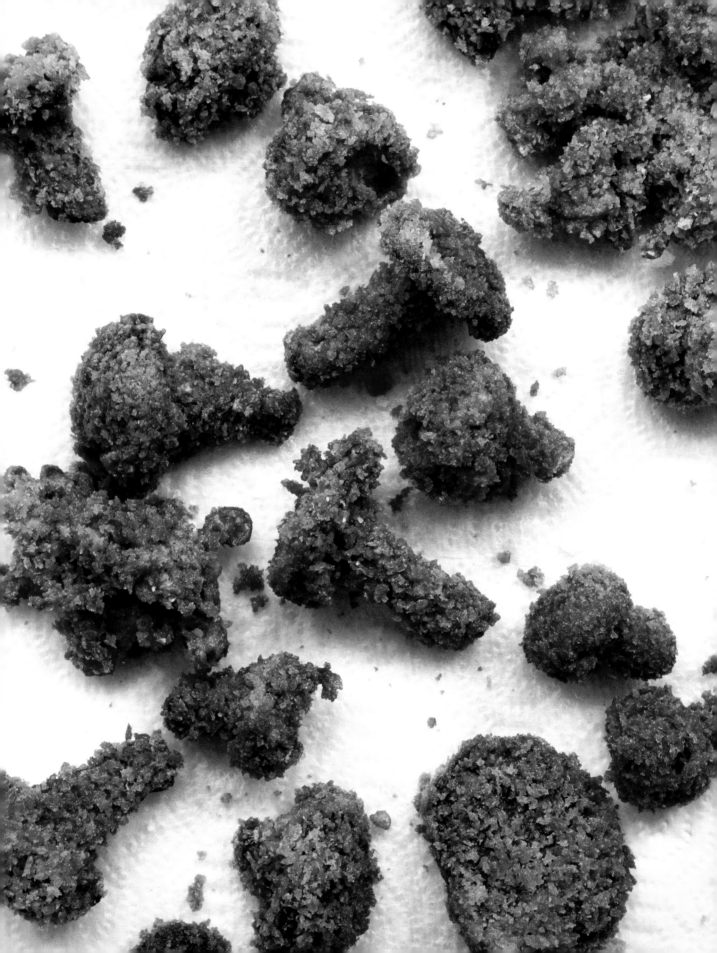

THC

9.5 mg per ½ cup aioli;
37.8 mg total recipe

Fried Mixed Mushrooms

Iliana Regan/Elizabeth

Yield: 4 servings and 2 cups aioli

Aioli

2 heads garlic

2 tablespoons freshly squeezed lemon juice

2 teaspoons kosher salt

4 egg yolks

1 tablespoon water

2 tablespoons flower-infused canola oil (see page 64)

½ cup plus 2 tablespoons canola oil

Mushrooms

¾ cup acorn flour

½ cup rye flour

⅓ cup all-purpose flour

Kosher salt

1 teaspoon freshly ground black pepper

4 large eggs

1½ cups panko (Japanese bread crumbs)

1 pound mixed mushrooms (such as shiitake, chanterelles, and button), stemmed if necessary and halved or broken into 2-inch pieces

2 tablespoons canola oil, plus more as needed

4 tablespoons unsalted butter, plus more as needed

Maldon sea salt for finishing

Yes, we know. Acorn flour is a big ask of anyone. You do have a few options, however. You can either go full prepper and process and mill acorns that you hunt and gather yourself; you can score some acorn flour off the internet; or, tbh, you can just use all rye flour. That said, taking the trouble to source acorn flour is totally worth it, as this dish, from consummate cool-person Iliana Regan of Chicago's Elizabeth, radiates the kind of earthy vibes that will make you want to eat it in the middle of a mossy forest.

To make the aioli: Heat the oven to 400°F.

Peel away the loose, papery outer skins from the garlic, leaving the heads intact. Wrap the garlic in aluminum foil and roast until a center clove is completely soft when pierced with a paring knife, about 40 minutes. Remove from the oven, unwrap, let cool, and then separate the cloves.

Squeeze the base of each clove to release the garlic from its papery sheath, dropping the garlic into a blender. Add the lemon juice, salt, egg yolks, and water and process for a few seconds until blended. With the motor running, very slowly drizzle in the infused canola oil. Once the mixture begins to thicken, add the regular canola oil in a thin, slow stream until all of the oil is incorporated and the aioli is smooth and thick. Transfer to an airtight container and store in the refrigerator for up to 2 weeks.

To make the mushrooms: In a medium bowl, whisk together all three flours, 1 tablespoon kosher salt, and the pepper. In a second medium bowl, whisk the eggs until blended. Put the panko in a third bowl.

continued

Fried Mixed Mushrooms, *continued*

Working in small batches, dust the mushrooms in the flour mixture, shaking off the excess, then dip them into the eggs, allowing the excess to drip off. Finally, dredge them in the panko, coating them evenly and shaking off the excess. Set aside on a large plate.

Line a second large plate with paper towels.

In a large cast-iron skillet over medium-high heat, warm the canola oil and butter. When the butter begins to bubble, add the mushrooms, working in batches to avoid crowding, and cook, flipping them once and sprinkling them with kosher salt, until browned all over, about 3 minutes total. Now, tilt the pan toward you, collect the buttery cooking fat in a spoon, and baste the mushrooms, coating their sides and crevices. Once the mushrooms are well browned, using a slotted spoon, transfer them to the prepared plate. Season the mushrooms with Maldon salt and serve warm with the aioli.

THC

2 mg per sandwich;
16 mg total recipe

With infused butter:
16.7 mg per sandwich;
501 mg total recipe

Collard Greens

4 tablespoons flower-infused butter (see page 68)

¼ cup minced fresh garlic

½ cup red wine vinegar

½ cup rice vinegar

½ cup granulated sugar

1 tablespoon Creole seasoning (we recommend Zatarain's brand)

1 tablespoon Korean red pepper powder (gochugaru)

1½ teaspoons kosher salt

1½ teaspoons freshly ground black pepper

½ cup water

2 pounds collard greens, stemmed and leaves chopped

Coleslaw

4 cups firmly packed thinly sliced green cabbage

¼ cup plus 2 tablespoons mayonnaise (we recommend Duke's brand)

2 tablespoons thinly sliced white onion

1 tablespoon distilled white vinegar

Kosher salt and freshly ground black pepper

The Collard Green Melt

Mason Hereford/Turkey and the Wolf
Yield: 8 sandwiches

Okay, so this isn't a salad. And it's not really a vegetable side, either. But it's so fucking good that it belongs here anyway. Dreamed up by Mason Hereford, a veteran of fine-dining kitchens who pitched it all to open Turkey and the Wolf (a chill sandwich spot in New Orleans), this sandwich is basically a cross between a club sandwich and a Reuben, with the addition of a mountain of greens (braised with more green). Your only job is to fit its layers of collard greens, coleslaw, Russian dressing, melted cheese, and rye bread into your mouth. You'll need to tap a Korean market (or shop online) for the red pepper powder, as no substitute will do.

Diluting ¼ cup of infused butter into 2 cups of potlikker results in a THC dose of approximately 2 mg per 1 tablespoon of liquid. Since most of the likker remains in the stockpot and not on a sandwich, the cannabis is being used to flavor the collard greens and most of the psychoactivity is left behind in the likker. Reserve the leftover likker to make a vegetable soup, or alternatively use the optional infused butter to toast the bread.

To cook the collard greens: In a large, heavy stockpot over medium heat, warm the infused butter. Add the garlic and cook, stirring occasionally, until fragrant and cooked through, about 2 minutes. Add both vinegars, the sugar, Creole seasoning, red pepper powder, salt, black pepper, and water and stir well. Cook, stirring occasionally, to allow the flavors to meld and develop, about 10 minutes.

Add the greens to the stockpot by the handful, waiting for each addition to wilt before adding the next. When all of the collards are added, cook, uncovered, over medium-low heat, stirring occasionally, until the greens are incredibly tender, 2 to 3 hours. Remove from the heat, let the collards cool in their potlikker, and then reserve until ready to prepare the sandwiches. (Store in a covered container in the refrigerator for up to 5 days.)

continued

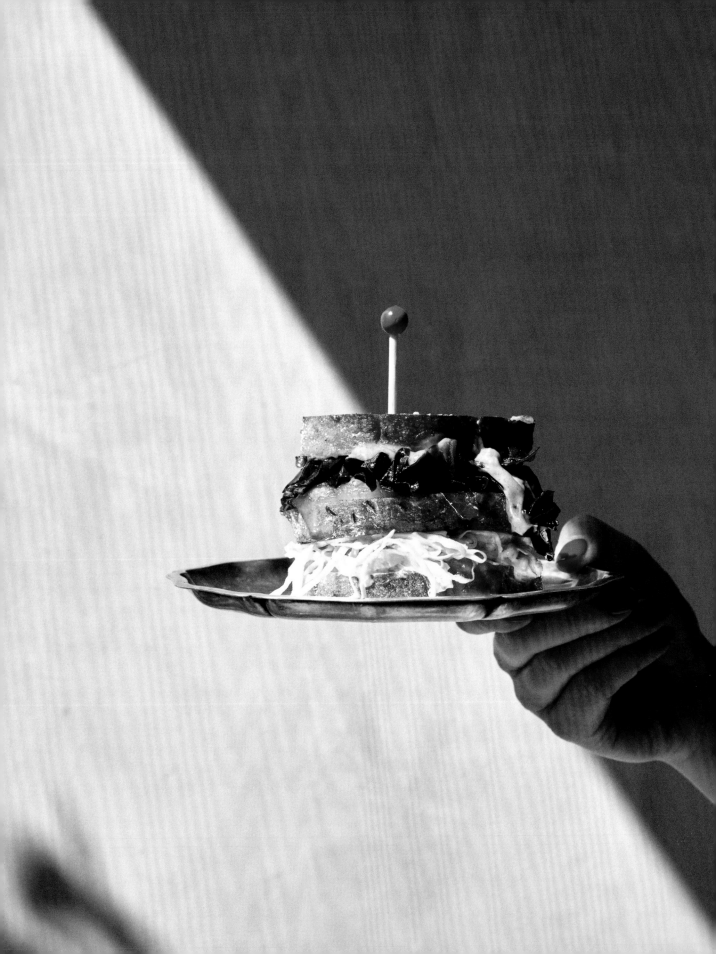

The Collard Green Melt, *continued*

Russian Dressing

¼ cup coarsely chopped hot pickled cherry peppers

¼ cup mayonnaise (we recommend Duke's brand)

¾ teaspoon ketchup

½ teaspoon Korean red pepper powder (gochugaru)

¼ teaspoon hot sauce (we recommend Crystal brand)

⅛ teaspoon smoked paprika

Kosher salt and freshly ground black pepper

8 tablespoons unsalted butter or flower-infused butter (see page 68), at room temperature

24 thin slices rye bread with caraway seeds

16 thick slices Swiss cheese

To make the coleslaw: In a large bowl, combine the cabbage, mayonnaise, onion, and vinegar and season with salt and pepper. Using your hands, massage the cabbage to break it down in the mayonnaise until it is reduced to about one-fourth of its original volume. Taste and adjust the seasoning if needed, then cover and refrigerate until ready to use. (Store in a covered container in the refrigerator for up to 1 day.)

To make the Russian dressing: In a small bowl, stir together the cherry peppers, mayonnaise, ketchup, red pepper powder, hot sauce, and paprika, mixing well. Season with salt and black pepper. Set aside.

Using ½ tablespoon butter per slice, brush butter on both sides of three bread slices. Warm a stove-top nonstick griddle or a large nonstick sauté pan over medium heat. Add the bread slices and toast on the first side until golden, about 1½ minutes. Flip the slices and top two of them with a cheese slice. Allow the cheese to melt fully, covering the slices with a pot lid to facilitate the melting process.

While the bread is toasting, in a sauté pan over medium heat, warm about 1 cup of the collards and about ¼ cup of potlikker.

Place a handful of coleslaw on a cheese-up slice of rye bread. Place the second piece of cheese-up bread on top of the coleslaw. Spoon the warm collard greens on top of the second cheese-up slice, leaving some potlikker behind (too much liquid will make the sandwich soggy). Dress the third slice of rye with a liberal slather of Russian dressing and place it, dressing-side down, on top of the collards. Cut the sandwich in half and serve immediately. Repeat to make the remaining sandwiches the same way.

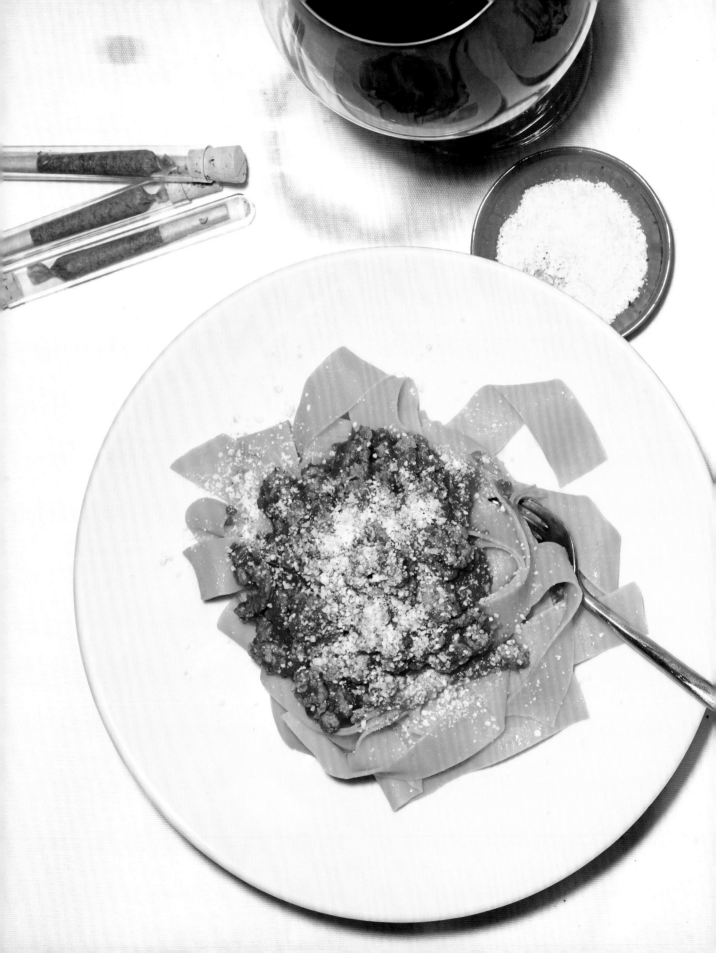

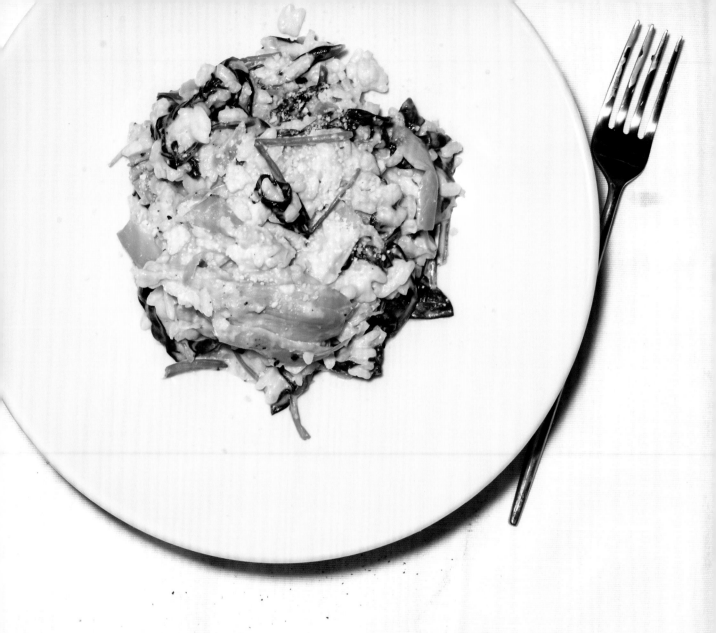

Pasta & Grains

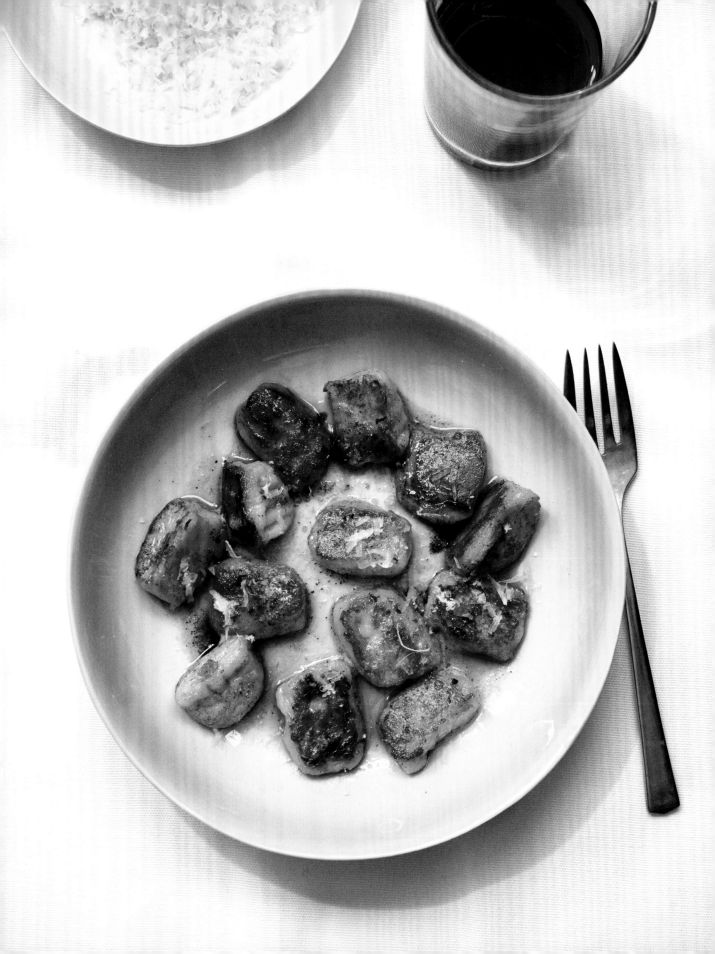

THC
11.5 mg per serving,
46 mg total recipe

Brown Butter Gnocchi

Aurora Leveroni (aka Nonna Marijuana)

Yield: 4 servings

Gnocchi

1½ pounds russet potatoes

1 tablespoon flower-infused olive oil (see page 64)

1 large egg, lightly beaten

½ teaspoon kosher salt

¾ cup all-purpose flour, plus more for dusting

Brown Butter

¾ cup unsalted butter

¼ cup weed-infused brown butter (see page 68), at room temperature

Kosher salt and freshly ground black pepper

Grated Parmesan cheese for serving

Aurora Leveroni is the ninety-four-year-old mother of legendary cannabis crusader Valerie Leveroni Corral, cofounder of the Wo/Men's Alliance for Medical Marijuana (WAMM) in Santa Cruz, California. Known fondly as "Nonna Marijuana," Aurora Leveroni focuses on creating infused food for the patients who need it most. These pillowy gnocchi are dosed in equal amounts with weed and love, Italian grandma–style. If you don't have a ricer (a metal basket with a perforated base through which the cooked potatoes are passed, yielding smooth, fluffy mashed potatoes), you can grate the potatoes on the large holes of a box grater, but you should probably get a ricer if you want the fluffiest-possible gnocchi.

There are a few ways to go about dosing this dish. Using the entire recipe of weed-infused brown butter adds a lot of flavor and more than 100 milligrams of THC. If each diner can handle a dose of 25 milligrams, that's probably the move. For a lower dose, do as this recipe directs and dilute ¼ cup infused brown butter with ¾ cup regular brown butter. Or you can rely solely on the weed-infused olive oil to get you high and use regular brown butter for dressing the gnocchi.

To make the gnocchi: In a medium saucepan over high heat, combine the potatoes with water to cover generously and bring to a boil. Adjust the heat to maintain a gentle boil and cook until soft when tested with a knife, 30 to 35 minutes. Drain the potatoes, let cool just until they can be handled, then peel and discard the skins.

Pass the potatoes through a ricer held over a large bowl, taking care to remove any lumps. Add the infused olive oil, egg, and salt and stir to combine. Then add the flour, a few spoonfuls at a time, mixing it in with your hands until all of the flour has been added and is evenly moistened and the dough begins to clump together. Knead the dough in the bowl until it is smooth, soft, and a little sticky. This should take no more than a minute or two.

continued

Brown Butter Gnocchi, *continued*

Line a large baking sheet with parchment paper and dust the paper with flour.

Divide the dough into four equal pieces. Transfer one piece to a lightly floured work surface and, using your palms, roll the dough into a long rope about ¾ inch in diameter. Using a sharp knife, cut the rope crosswise into 1-inch pieces. Make an indentation in the center of each piece by pressing your thumb into it while rolling it over the back of a fork. Transfer the finished gnocchi, in a single layer and not touching, to the prepared baking sheet and cover with a kitchen towel. Repeat to shape gnocchi with the remaining dough. (The gnocchi will keep, covered with the towel, in the refrigerator until ready to cook or up to 24 hours. Alternatively, you can freeze the gnocchi on the baking sheet, then transfer them to ziplock plastic freezer bags and freeze for up to 3 months; add them to the boiling water directly from the freezer.)

To make the brown butter: In a large skillet over medium-high, melt the unsalted butter. Cook for about 4 minutes, until the butter turns a light brown and has a nutty smell. Remove from the heat and stir in the infused butter. Set aside and keep warm until you have your gnocchi cooked.

Bring a large pot of generously salted water to a boil. Add the gnocchi and cook until they float to the surface, 3 to 4 minutes. Using a slotted spoon, transfer the gnocchi to the skillet with the brown butter and toss to combine. Season with salt and pepper and serve with Parmesan on the side.

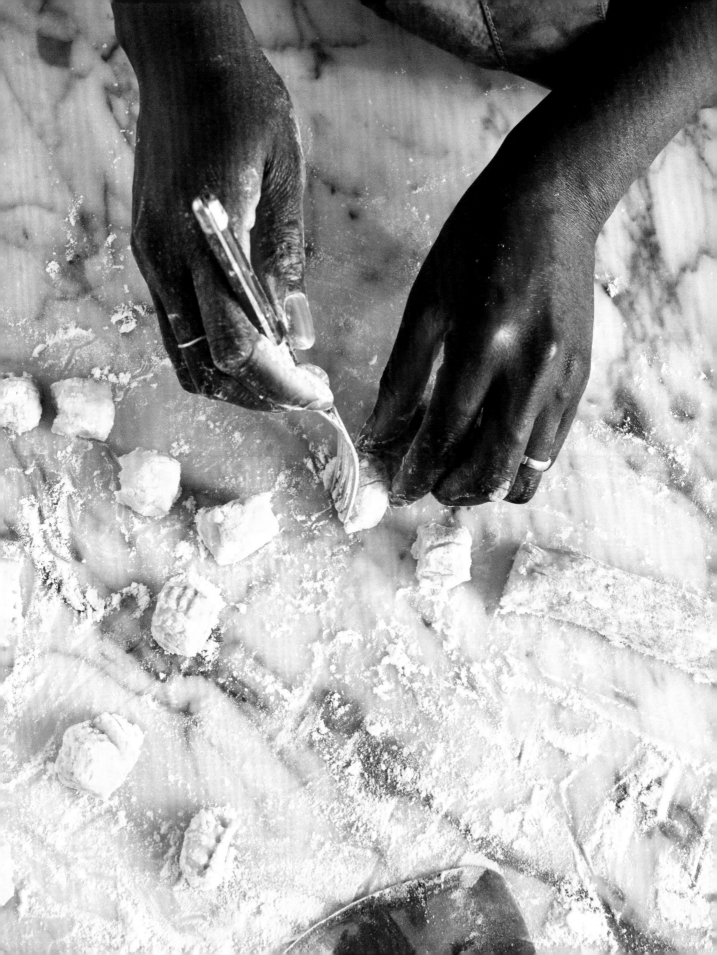

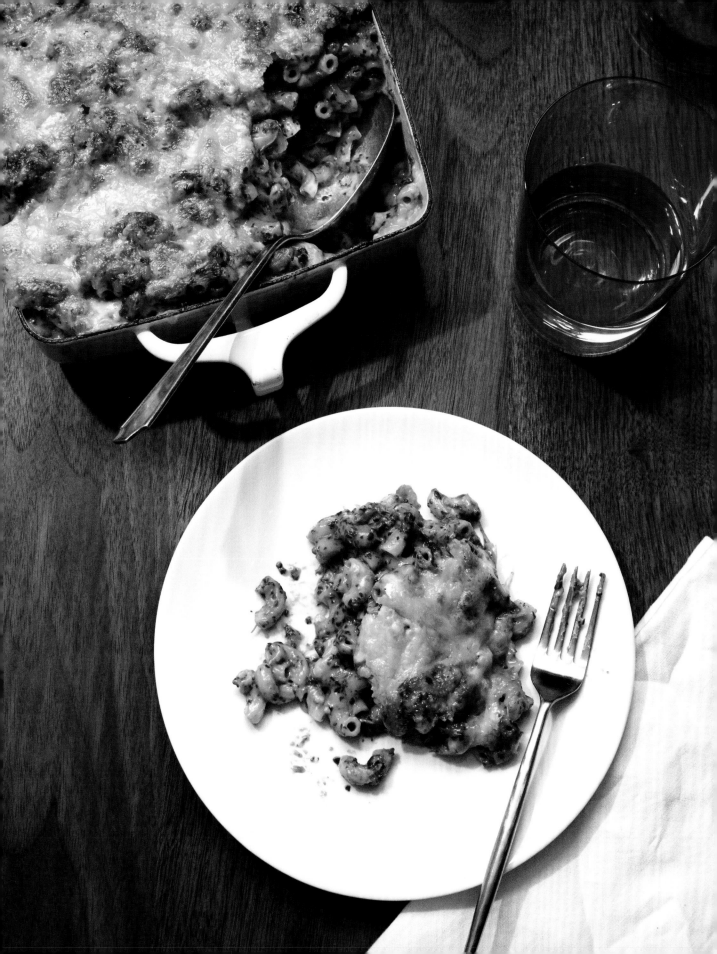

THC

5.5 mg per serving;
33.4 mg total recipe

Green Mac and Cheese

MUNCHIES Test Kitchen

Yield: 6 servings

Two 5-ounce packages
baby spinach

1 cup firmly packed fresh
flat-leaf parsley leaves

1 cup firmly packed fresh
basil leaves

1 cup grated Parmesan cheese

1 garlic clove

3½ cups whole milk

2 tablespoons flower-infused
butter (see page 68)

2 tablespoons unsalted butter

⅓ cup all-purpose flour

3 cups grated white cheddar
cheese

Kosher salt and freshly ground
black pepper

1 pound elbow macaroni

A healthy amount of baby spinach and a healthier amount of infused butter turn this incredibly cheesy comfort-food classic green.

In the bowl of a food processor, combine the spinach, parsley, basil, Parmesan, and garlic and pulse until chunky. Add ½ cup of the milk and process until smooth. Set aside.

In a 6-quart saucepan over medium-high heat, melt both butters. Add the flour and cook, stirring constantly, until thick and smooth, about 2 minutes. Continuing to stir constantly, add the remaining 3 cups milk and then cook, stirring occasionally, until thick and creamy, 8 to 10 minutes. Add half of the cheddar and stir until melted. Season with salt and pepper.

Meanwhile, bring a large pot of salted water to a boil. Add the macaroni and cook, stirring occasionally, until al dente, according to package directions.

While the macaroni cooks, heat the broiler.

When the pasta is ready, drain it and add to the cheese sauce along with the spinach mixture. Stir to coat the macaroni evenly. Spread the macaroni mixture in a broiler-safe 9 by 13-inch baking dish, then top evenly with the remaining cheddar. Set the baking dish on a baking sheet and place under the broiler until the top is golden brown and macaroni and cheese is bubbling, 5 to 7 minutes. Let cool for 10 minutes before serving.

THC

7.5 mg per serving;
45 mg total recipe

Peanut Butter Noodles

MUNCHIES Test Kitchen
Yield: 6 servings

1 pound spaghetti

2 red bell peppers, seeded and thinly sliced lengthwise

1 English cucumber, halved lengthwise, seeded, and thinly sliced crosswise

½ cup crushed roasted peanuts

3 green onions, white and tender green parts, thinly sliced

⅔ cup Homemade Peanut Butter (page 232)

⅓ cup soy sauce

¼ cup firmly packed light brown sugar

⅓ cup water

Fresh cilantro leaves for garnish

These super-easy noodles are like a 1990s Chinese-takeout throwback, in all the best ways. Infused peanut butter lives its best possible life in the sauce here, but if you don't have any on hand, regular peanut butter with a little infused oil stirred in works just as well.

Bring a large pot of generously salted water to a boil. Add the spaghetti and cook, stirring occasionally, until al dente, according to package directions. Drain the pasta, rinse under cool running water, drain again, and transfer to a large bowl. Add the bell peppers, cucumber, peanuts, and green onions and toss to mix.

Meanwhile, in a small bowl, whisk together the peanut butter, soy sauce, brown sugar, and water until evenly incorporated into a sauce.

Add the sauce to the pasta and toss to coat the noodles and vegetables evenly. Transfer to a serving bowl and garnish with cilantro. Serve immediately.

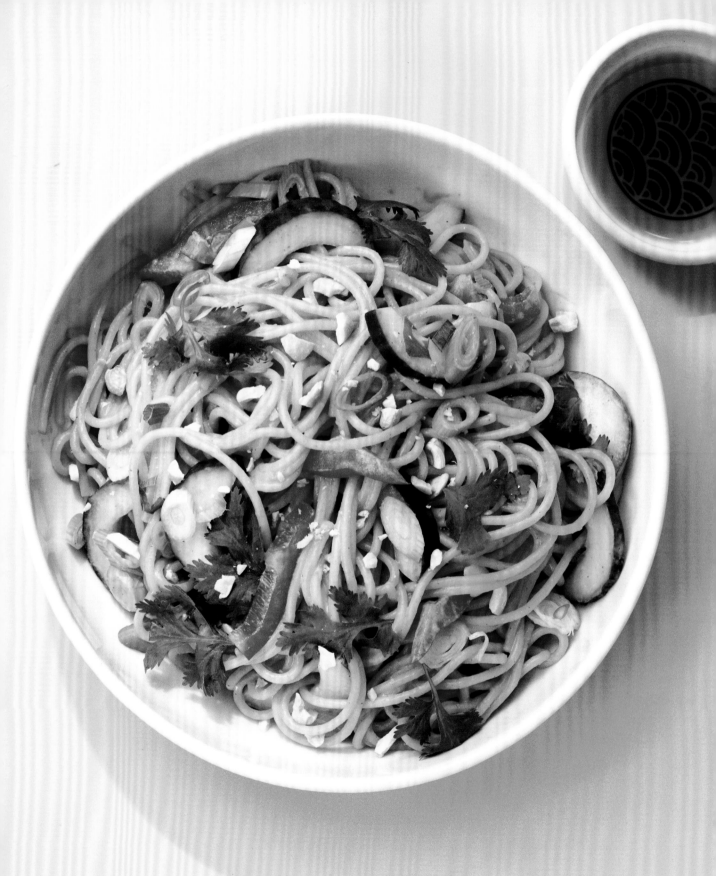

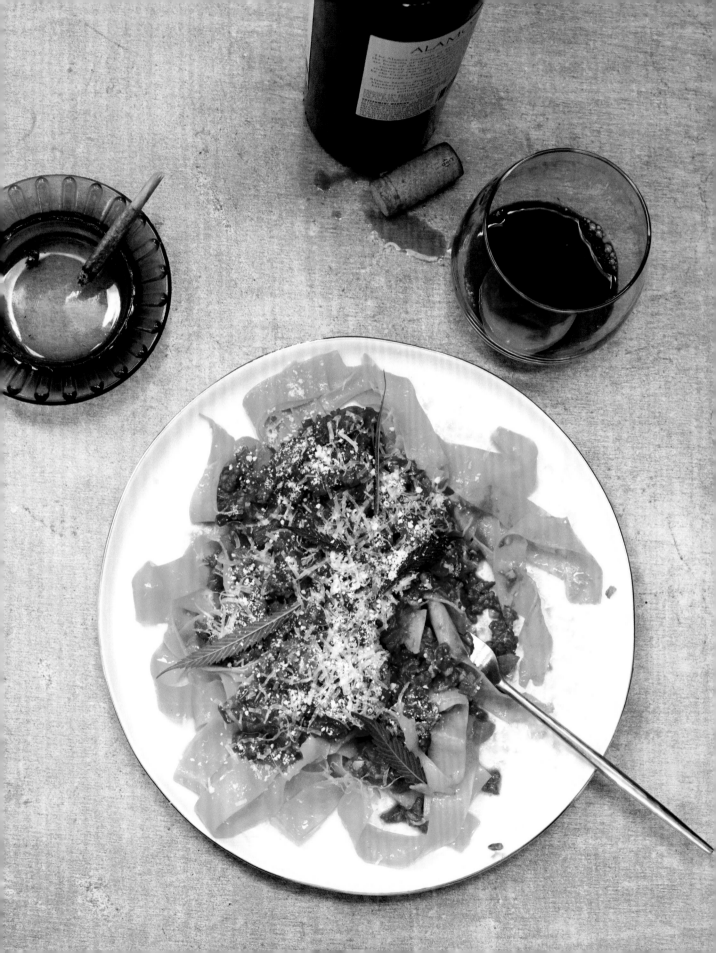

THC
5.5 mg per serving;
33.4 mg total recipe

With infused cream:
16.5 mg per serving;
100.3 mg total recipe

Sausage Pappardelle Bolognese

MUNCHIES Test Kitchen

Yield: 6 servings

2 tablespoons olive oil

2 tablespoons flower-infused butter (see page 68)

6 garlic cloves, finely chopped

1 carrot, peeled and finely chopped

1 celery stalk, finely chopped

1 small yellow onion, finely chopped

1 pound weed-infused sweet Italian sausage (see page 241), casings removed

½ teaspoon red pepper flakes

Kosher salt and freshly ground black pepper

2 tablespoons tomato paste

½ cup dry red wine

One 28-ounce can whole tomatoes in juice, crushed by hand

¼ cup plus 2 tablespoons heavy cream

2 tablespoons weed-infused cream (see page 72; optional)

1 pound dried pappardelle

Grated Parmesan cheese for serving

Vanessa Says: Always follow your nose when picking varieties. In a Bolognese, Girl Scout Cookies or a peppery Bubba Kush will add a nice flavor to the overall dish.

The infused sausage works magic in this Italian-American dinner-table staple, which comes together much more quickly than a classic Bolognese sauce. If you're not up to at-home charcuterie, use store-bought Italian sausage instead and dose the final dish with a drizzle of infused olive oil (see page 64) or a dollop of infused ricotta (see page 233). Slivered fan leaves add a decorative finish.

In a large saucepan over medium-high heat, warm the olive oil and infused butter. Add the garlic, carrot, celery, and onion and cook, stirring often, until golden, 8 to 10 minutes. Add the sausage and red pepper flakes, season with salt and pepper, and cook, stirring and breaking up the meat with a wooden spoon, until the sausage is crumbly, has lost its raw red color, and has browned, about 8 minutes.

Add the tomato paste to the pan and cook, stirring, for about 2 minutes. Pour in the wine, stir well to dislodge any browned bits on the pan bottom, and boil gently until reduced by half, about 3 minutes. Add the tomatoes and bring to a boil. Lower the heat to maintain a simmer and cook, stirring occasionally, until the sauce is thick, about 6 minutes longer. Stir in the heavy cream and infused cream (if using) and simmer for 3 minutes to blend the flavors, then keep warm.

Meanwhile, bring a large pot of generously salted water to a boil. Add the pappardelle and cook, stirring occasionally, until al dente, according to package directions. Drain the pasta, toss with the sauce, and serve immediately. Pass the Parmesan at the table.

THC
6.2 mg per serving;
50 mg total recipe

With cannabis flower:
6.3 mg per serving;
51.5 mg total recipe

Spinach and Artichoke Dip Risotto

MUNCHIES Test Kitchen

Yield: 8 servings

6 cups chicken stock

6 cannabis fan leaves (optional)

5 whole black peppercorns

1 rosemary sprig

1 thyme sprig

0.5 gram cannabis flower, freshly ground (optional)

3 tablespoons flower-infused butter (see page 68)

1 large yellow onion, diced

2 cups Arborio rice

1 cup dry white wine

One 5-ounce package baby spinach

½ cup grated Parmesan cheese

1 cup cream cheese, at room temperature, cut into chunks

Two 13½-ounce cans quartered artichoke hearts, drained

Kosher salt and freshly ground black pepper

Here's your favorite dip turned into a risotto, because we're classy like that. If you want to take it to the next level, a little extra freshly ground cannabis flower infused into the stock wouldn't hurt. Using cannabis as a spice adds extra flavor to this dish and works with the spinach without any further potency. You don't have to dip tortilla chips into it to keep it true to its dip origins. But, then, you also don't *not* have to.

In a saucepan over medium-low heat, warm the chicken stock to a simmer. While the stock is heating, put the cannabis leaves (if using), peppercorns, rosemary, thyme, and, if you're feeling flush, cannabis flower on a piece of cheesecloth, tie together the corners to make a sachet, and add the sachet to the stock. Keep the stock warm over very low heat.

In a 6-quart saucepan over medium-high heat, melt the infused butter. Add the onion and cook, stirring often, until golden, 6 to 8 minutes. Add the rice and cook, stirring occasionaly, until lightly toasted, about 4 minutes. Pour in the wine and cook, stirring constantly, until evaporated, about 2 minutes. Add ½ cup of the warm stock and cook, stirring, until it has been absorbed, about 2 minutes. Continue adding stock, ½ cup at a time, stirring and cooking until it is absorbed before adding more, until the rice is tender and creamy. The total cooking time will be about 22 minutes.

Stir half of the spinach into the pan, allow the leaves to wilt completely, and then stir in the remaining spinach. Add the Parmesan, cream cheese, and artichoke hearts and cook, stirring, until the cheeses have melted and the artichoke hearts are heated through. Season with salt and pepper and serve immediately.

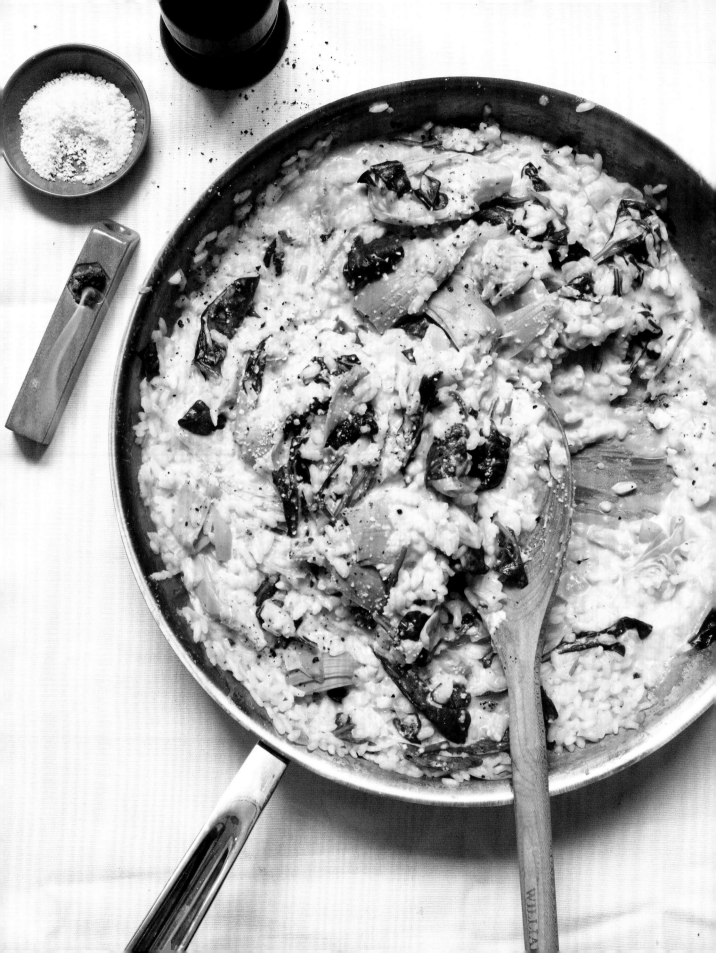

THC

5.5 mg per serving;
33.4 mg total recipe

With kief: 9.2 mg per serving;
55.6 mg total recipe

Chicken Rice (Riz a Djaj)

Rebecca Merhej/Love & Salt

Yield: 6 servings

2 whole chicken breasts

1 cinnamon stick, ½ teaspoon ground cinnamon, plus more for sprinkling

Kosher salt

1 pound lean ground lamb

2 tablespoons flower-infused butter (see page 68)

½ teaspoon freshly ground black pepper

½ teaspoon ground allspice

0.5 gram raw kief (optional)

1½ cups long-grain white rice, rinsed and drained

1 tablespoon vegetable oil

½ cup sliced or slivered almonds

½ cup pine nuts

½ cup plain whole-milk yogurt

Rebecca Merhej from L.A.'s Love & Salt made us this wildly satisfying chicken-lamb-rice bowl—just exactly what you want to curl up with at the end of a long day. It's what Lebanese grandma comfort-food would look like if your Lebanese grandma had access to high-end green and a generous hand with the seasoning.

Put the chicken breasts in a medium saucepan; add water to cover by 1 inch, the cinnamon stick, and 1 teaspoon salt; and bring to a boil over medium-high heat. Turn the heat to a gentle simmer, cover, and cook until the chicken is opaque throughout and tender, 20 to 30 minutes. Remove from the heat and transfer the chicken to a shallow bowl. Strain the cooking liquid through a fine-mesh strainer and reserve.

When the chicken is cool enough to handle, remove and discard the skin and bones and then shred the meat. Return the chicken to the bowl, add a splash of the reserved cooking liquid, and set aside.

Place a dry large skillet over medium heat. Add the lamb and cook, stirring and breaking up the meat with a wooden spoon, until the lamb has lost its raw red color and is browned, about 10 minutes. Stir in the infused butter, 1½ teaspoons salt, the pepper, allspice, ground cinnamon, and kief (if using), mixing well. Cover and cook for 10 minutes, stirring often to prevent sticking.

Add the rice and 2½ cups of the reserved cooking liquid to the skillet, stir well, cover, and bring to a boil. Lower the heat to a steady simmer and cook, covered, until the liquid is absorbed and the rice is tender, about 20 minutes.

While the rice cooks, line a plate with a paper towel.

In a medium skillet over medium heat, warm the vegetable oil. Add the almonds and pine nuts and toast, tossing or stirring constantly to prevent burning, until golden, about 4 minutes. Using a slotted spoon, transfer the nuts to the prepared plate to drain.

In a small bowl, stir together the yogurt and a pinch of salt, cover, and refrigerate until ready to use.

When the rice mixture is ready, fluff it with a fork, then fold in half of the almonds and pine nuts. Scoop the rice onto a serving platter and top with shredded chicken. Garnish with the remaining pine nuts and almonds, sprinkle with a little ground cinnamon, and finish with dollops of the yogurt.

Pro Tip: The nutty, cinnamon-y flavors here work well with earthy raw kief and spicy weed strains like Mazar Kush, Hindu Kush, Kosher Kush, Hash Plant, and Red Dragon. If you're interested in significantly increasing the THC dose, toast your kief in a 240°F oven for 30 minutes to decarboxylate it and activate more THC (see page 55).

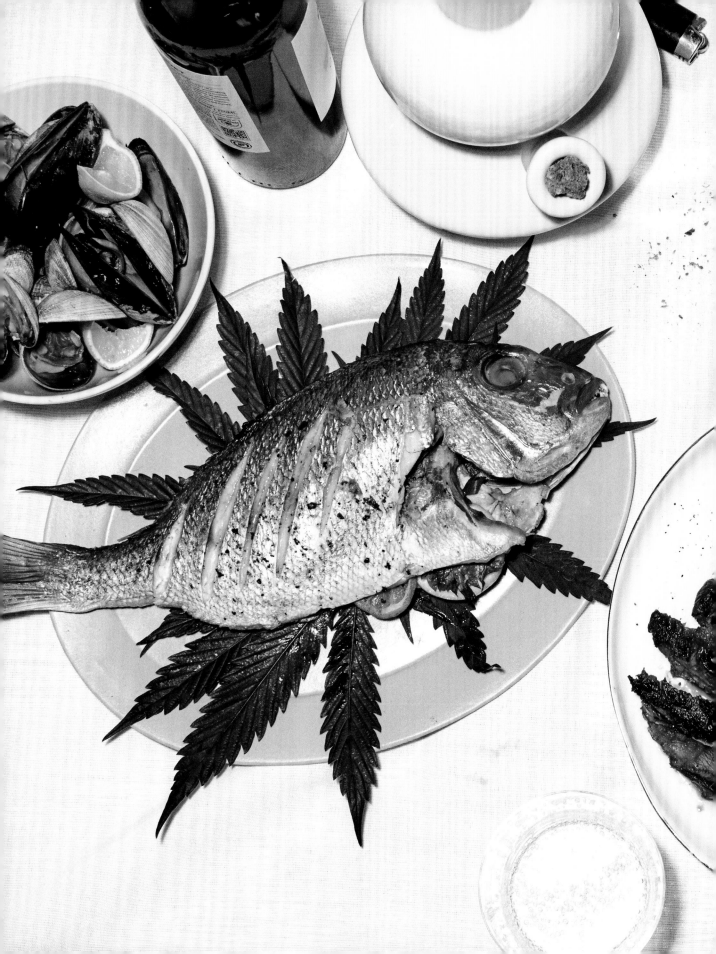

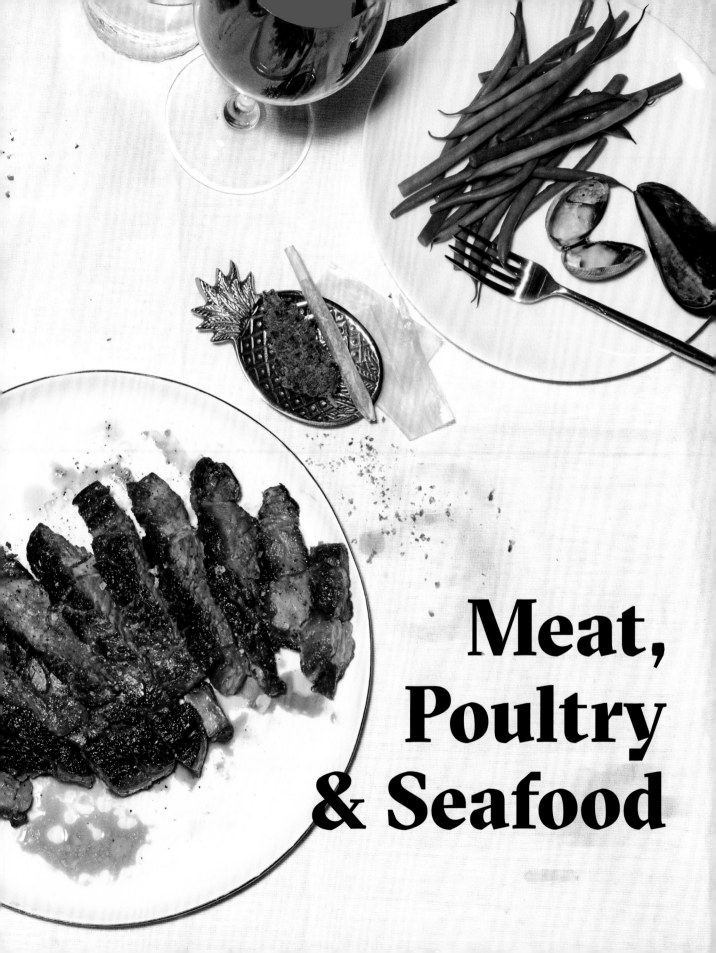

Meat,
Poultry
& Seafood

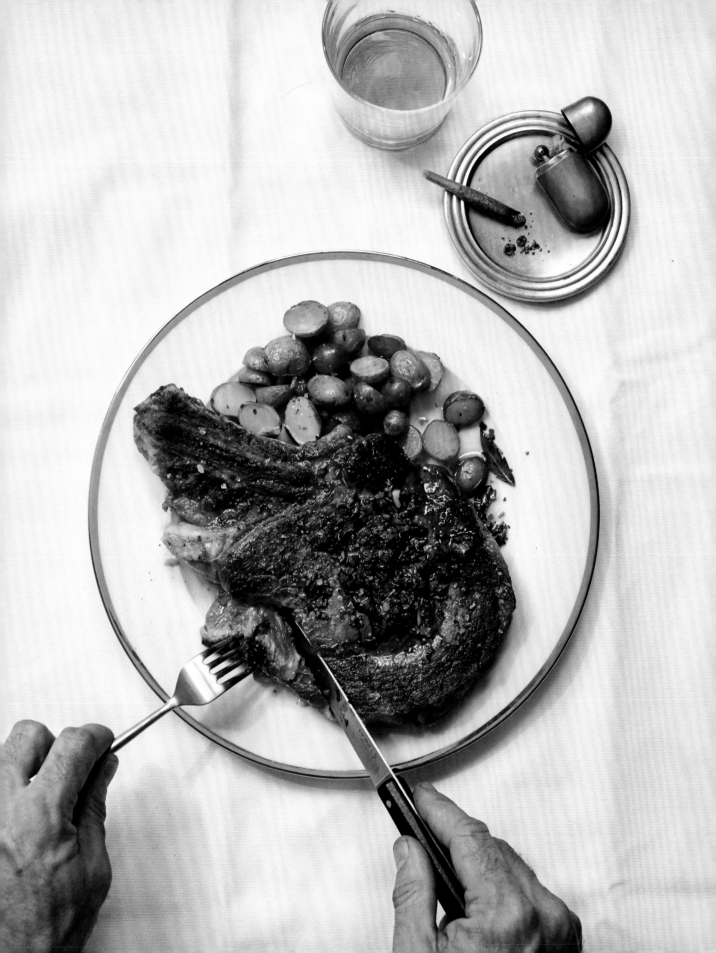

THC
5.2 mg per serving;
10.4 mg total recipe

With infused butter:
11.2 mg per serving;
16.4 mg total recipe

Rib-Eye with Weed Chimichurri

Tim Milojevich

Yield: 2 servings

2 bone-in rib-eye steaks

Kosher salt and freshly ground black pepper

Chimichurri

Leaves from 1 bunch flat-leaf parsley, finely chopped

8 cannabis fan leaves, finely chopped (optional)

3 tablespoons red wine vinegar

1 tablespoon kosher salt

3 garlic cloves, minced

2 teaspoons dried oregano

1 teaspoon red pepper flakes

1 tablespoon flower-infused olive oil (see page 64)

¾ cup plus 3 tablespoons olive oil

2 tablespoons kief-infused butter (see page 68; optional)

Pot leaves don't get nearly enough credit. Sure, they're basically the universal symbol for weed, but there's also room for them in places that aren't necklaces, flags, and cheesy tie-dyed T-shirts. Like this tangy chimichurri from private chef Tim Milojevich, where their vegetal notes shine alongside parsley and red pepper. The leaves themselves aren't psychoactive but the olive oil they're mixed with is, and there's plenty of it.

Rub the steaks with a generous amount of salt and pepper. Let rest, uncovered, in the refrigerator for at least 10 hours or up to overnight. Remove the steaks from the refrigerator 2 hours before cooking to allow them to come to room temperature.

To make the chimichurri: In a medium bowl, combine the parsley, cannabis leaves (if using), vinegar, salt, garlic, oregano, red pepper flakes, and infused olive oil and stir to mix well. Transfer to an air-tight container and store in the refrigerator for up to 2 days.

In a large cast-iron skillet over medium-high heat, warm the regular olive oil. Working with one rib-eye at a time, cook, flipping once, until well browned and cooked to desired doneness. The timing will depend on the thickness of the steak; a steak ¾ inch thick will take 8 to 10 minutes for medium-rare, or 135°F on an instant-read thermometer. Transfer the rib-eye to a cutting board and let rest for 10 minutes. Repeat with the remaining steak.

Cut the steaks against the grain into slices about ½ inch thick and transfer to individual plates. Serve topped with the infused butter, if desired, and accompanied with the chimichurri.

THC
4 mg per serving;
16.7 mg total recipe

Braised Short Ribs

The Publican

Yield: 4 servings

Short Ribs

3 pounds beef short ribs

Green Hatch chile powder for seasoning

Kosher salt

2 tablespoons vegetable oil

2 carrots, peeled and diced

2 celery stalks, diced

1 yellow onion, diced

2 thyme sprigs

1 bay leaf

2 cups red wine

8 cups beef stock

Polenta

4 cups whole milk, plus more as needed

1 cup coarse-grind polenta

1 tablespoon flower-infused butter (see page 68)

7 tablespoons unsalted butter

Kosher salt

The Publican in Chicago is basically a shrine to high-quality, farmhouse-style meat-and-potatoes eating—to say nothing of the butcher shop next door. These braised, chile-dusted short ribs are served on a bed of creamy weed polenta and finished with a briny, tangy sea bean salsa verde. (You can find Hatch chile powder and sea beans in a well-stocked grocery store.) If you have it, a little raw kief or CBD-infused salt on the short ribs along with the salsa verde wouldn't necessarily be a bad thing—why should the polenta have all the fun?

To prepare the short ribs: Season the ribs all over with chile powder and salt. Place on a rack set on a baking sheet and refrigerate, uncovered, for at least 8 hours or up to overnight.

Heat the oven to 325°F.

In a large, heavy saucepan over high heat, warm the vegetable oil. Working in batches, sear the ribs, turning them as needed to color evenly, until golden brown all over, 8 to 10 minutes. Transfer the ribs to a plate and set aside.

Add the carrots, celery, onion, thyme, and bay leaf to the fat remaining in the pan and cook over medium-high heat, stirring often, until the vegetables are slightly caramelized, about 7 minutes. Add the wine and bring to a boil, scraping up any browned bits on the pan bottom. Lower the heat to a steady simmer and let simmer until the wine is reduced by half, about 10 minutes. Return the ribs to the pan, pour in the beef stock, cover, and cook until the meat is tender when pierced with a fork and almost falling off the bone, 2½ to 3 hours.

To make the polenta: About 45 minutes before the ribs are ready, in a medium, heavy saucepan over medium heat, bring the milk to a simmer. Gradually add the polenta to the simmering milk while stirring constantly to prevent lumps from forming. Turn the heat to low and

continued

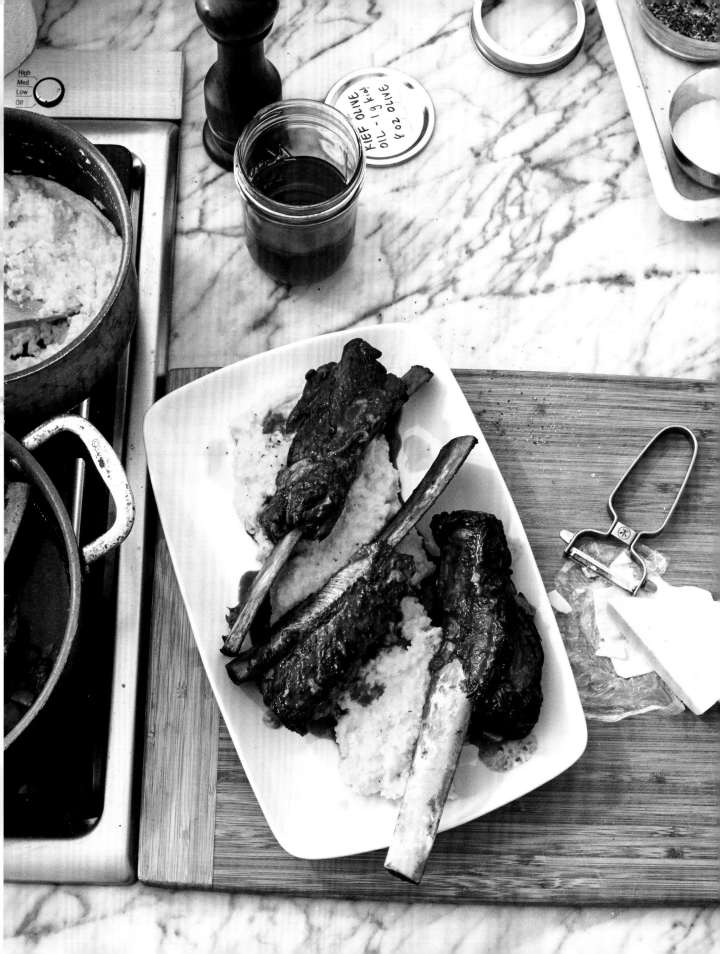

THC
5.2 mg per serving;
10.4 mg total recipe

Yogurt-Marinated Lamb

Erika Nakamura

Yield: 2 servings

⅓ cup olive oil

5 garlic cloves; 4 halved and
1 grated (optional)

4 thyme sprigs

2 rosemary sprigs

1 cup plain whole-milk
Greek yogurt

2 tablespoons red wine vinegar

Kosher salt and freshly ground
black pepper

1 rack of lamb (8 chops),
at room temperature

1 tablespoon flower-infused
olive oil (see page 64)

Lemon wedges for squeezing

Erika Nakamura is a butcher's butcher. She's spent a long stint at New York City's White Gold, along with partner Jocelyn Guest, and cofounded L.A.'s Lindy and Grundy—so it's no surprise that she'd come correct here. A grilled rack of lamb is one of those impressive-af dinner-party foods where no one needs to know how difficult it actually wasn't. Pair this with the tomato and stone fruit salad on page 120 and with a pinier, skunkier strain of cannabis, like an old-school Afghani or Shiva Senti, to bring out the herb notes in the lamb. Either strain would work just as well in the olive oil as it would in a joint beforehand.

In a small saucepan over medium-low heat, combine the olive oil, halved garlic, thyme, and rosemary; bring to a gentle simmer; and cook for about 15 minutes. Remove from the heat and let cool completely. Transfer to a large bowl and stir in the yogurt, vinegar, and grated garlic (if using). Season the marinade with salt and pepper.

Add the lamb to the marinade and turn to coat evenly. Cover and refrigerate for at least 8 hours or up to 24 hours.

Prepare a charcoal or gas grill for indirect-heat grilling.

Remove the lamb from the marinade, scraping off most of the marinade and being careful to remove any bits of herb, and bring to room temperature.

When the fire is ready, place the lamb rack, bone-side down, on the grill directly over the fire and cook until lightly browned, 3 to 4 minutes. Flip the lamb, placing it meat-side down over indirect heat, and cook to desired doneness, about 10 minutes for medium-rare or 125° to 130°F on an instant-read thermometer.

Transfer the lamb to a cutting board and let rest for about 10 minutes, then carve between the bones into individual chops. Divide among individual plates and drizzle with the infused olive oil and a squeeze of lemon juice. Serve immediately.

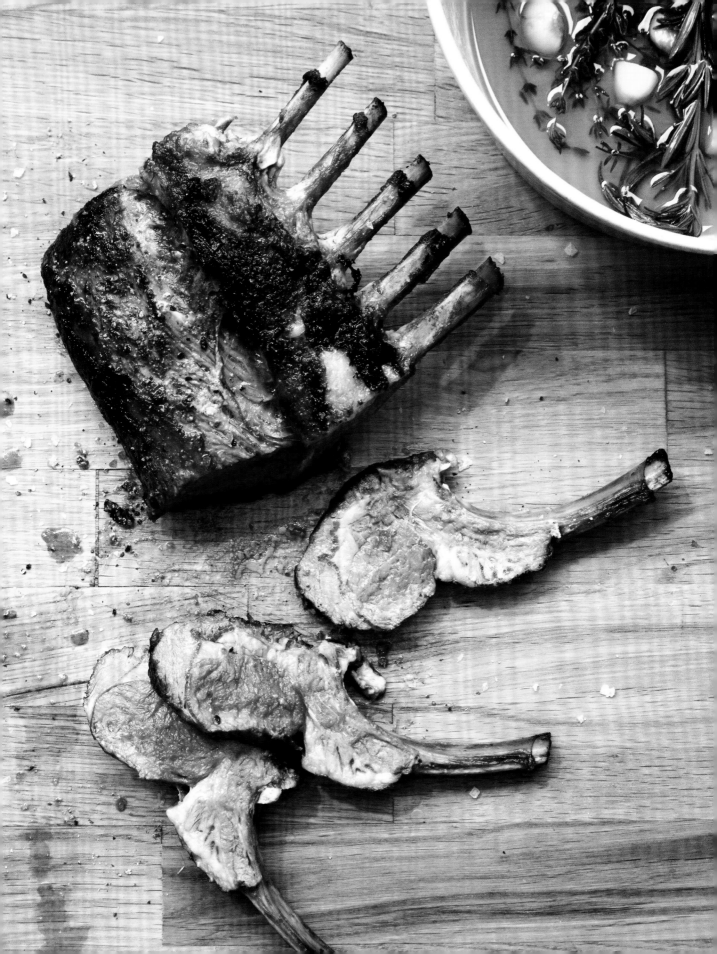

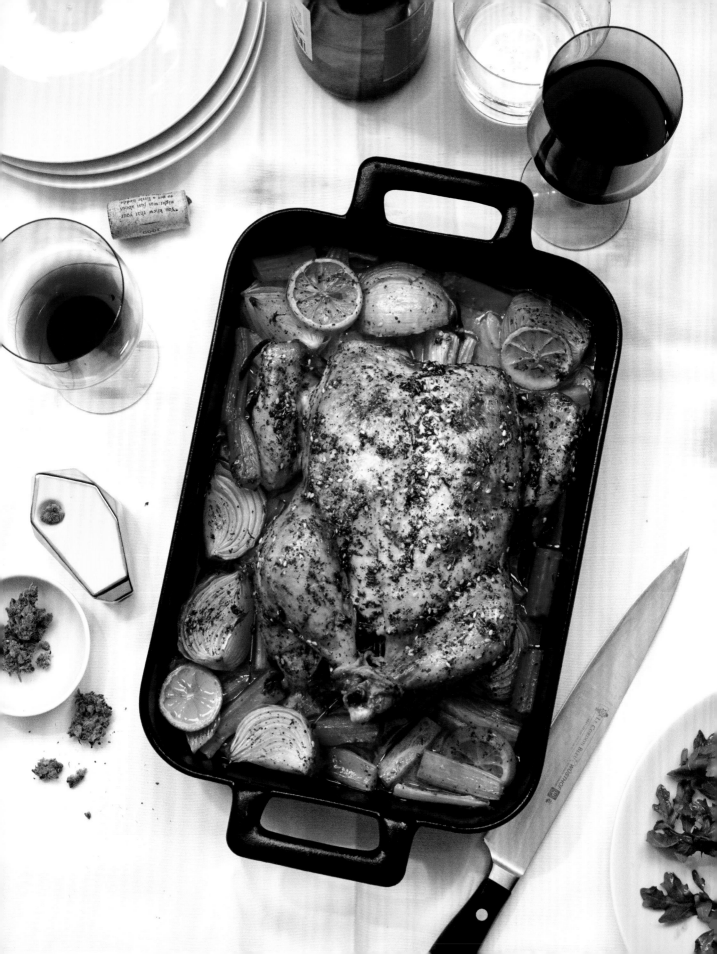

THC
5.7 mg per serving;
22.8 mg total recipe

Double-Lemon Roast Chicken

Joan Nathan

Yield: 4 servings

One 3- to 4-pound whole chicken

2 tablespoons flower-infused olive oil (see page 64)

Kosher salt and freshly ground black pepper

1 to 2 tablespoons za'atar

1 teaspoon ground sumac

1 preserved lemon (see page 228), halved and ½ diced

8 thyme sprigs

4 rosemary sprigs

2 sage sprigs

1 yellow onion, cut into about 8 pieces

2 lemons, thinly sliced into rounds

1 celery stalk, cut into 2-inch pieces

1 carrot, peeled and cut into 2-inch pieces

1 fennel bulb, trimmed and cut into 2-inch pieces

¾ cup dry white wine

Joan Nathan is basically the grand dame of Jewish home cooking. Even though she had never even seen weed in her life before coming on *Bong Appétit*, she was completely down to experiment. The result? This ultra-lemony roast chicken that uses both fresh lemons and preserved lemons to maximum advantage. Use a citrusy strain of herb, like Lemon Skunk, to round out the experience.

Heat the oven to 375°F.

Rub the chicken with the infused olive oil, then season with salt, pepper, as much of the za'atar as you like, and the sumac.

Place the chicken, breast-side up, in a 9 by 13-inch baking dish. Put the preserved lemon half and a sprig each of the thyme, rosemary, and sage in the cavity. Scatter the onion pieces, lemon slices, diced preserved lemon, celery, carrot, fennel, and remaining thyme, rosemary, and sage around the chicken. Pour in the wine.

Roast the chicken until golden brown and crispy and an instant-read thermometer inserted into the thickest part of the thigh away from bone registers 165°F, about 1¼ hours.

Remove the chicken from the oven, let rest for about 10 minutes, and then cut into eight pieces. Arrange the pieces on a platter and spoon the vegetables, preserved lemon and lemon slices, and pan juices over and around the chicken. Serve immediately.

THC
5.8 mg per serving;
34.9 mg total recipe

Korean Fried Chicken

Deuki Hong/Sunday Bird

Yield: 2 servings

Kimchi Ganja Salt

2 tablespoons onion powder

1 tablespoon garlic powder

1 tablespoon shrimp powder

1 teaspoon citric acid

1 teaspoon coconut sugar or granulated sugar

1 teaspoon ground ginger

1 gram cannabis flower, ground and decarboxylated (see page 55)

¼ cup kosher salt

Marinade

¼ cup olive oil

¼ cup soy sauce

3 tablespoons kosher salt

12 garlic cloves

1 yellow onion, quartered through the stem end

Grated zest and juice of 1 lemon

2 pounds chicken wings

1 cup cornstarch

Canola oil for frying

Batter

1 cup all-purpose flour

1 cup cornstarch

1 teaspoon baking powder

1 cup soju or vodka

1 cup water

Deuki Hong, chef at Sunday Bird in San Francisco, said he had never cooked with weed before he came on *Bong Appétit*. But after tasting his infused food, we're not sure we believe him. Between the killer kimchi fried rice he made on the show and these crispy, spicy Korean-style fried chicken wings, he's clearly some kind of weed savant. The kimchi ganja salt that tops these wings is a versatile addition to other dishes, too. You might use it to perk up (or mellow out) scrambled eggs, or fold it into softened butter for topping a grilled steak.

This recipe has a lot of steps and calls for some ingredients you might need to seek out via specialty grocery stores or (gasp) the internet. Citric acid, a sour-tasting powder found in the canning or spice section of markets, is a good example of an ingredient you'll probably need to hunt down. We promise the search is worth it.

To make the kimchi ganja salt: With a mortar and pestle, combine the onion powder, garlic powder, shrimp powder, citric acid, sugar, ginger, and cannabis flower and grind to a fine powder. Alternatively, combine the ingredients in a spice grinder and grind to a fine powder. Transfer the ground mixture to a small bowl, add the salt, and stir to combine. Transfer to an airtight container and store in the refrigerator for up to 3 months.

To make the marinade: In a blender, combine the olive oil, soy sauce, salt, garlic, onion, lemon zest, and lemon juice and process until smooth.

Poke holes all over the chicken wings with the tines of a fork. In a large bowl, toss the wings with the marinade until evenly coated. Cover and refrigerate for at least 2 hours or up to overnight.

Fit a baking sheet with a wire rack.

Remove the chicken wings from the marinade, allowing the excess to drip off, and place in a clean large bowl. Toss with the cornstarch, coating evenly, then transfer to the wire rack and let sit at room temperature for 30 minutes (this allows the cornstarch to hydrate and form a skin on the wings).

Vanessa Says: This is one of the rare occasions when you can grind decarboxylated flower with everything else in the salt blend, as it's getting paired with a fat that will help absorb it. Choose a spicy, earthy flower like Northern Lights or Kosher Kush; toasting brings out a nuttier flavor as well as activates the THC.

Pour the canola oil to a depth of 3 inches in a large, wide, heavy saucepan and heat to 350°F on a deep-frying (candy) thermometer. Line a plate with a double thickness of paper towel.

To make the batter: While the oil heats, in a medium bowl, combine the flour, cornstarch, baking powder, soju, and water and stir until the mixture has the consistency of watered-down glue.

Working in batches, dip the wings in the batter and let the excess drip off. Transfer the wings to the hot oil, a few at a time, and fry, turning as needed to color evenly, until golden brown and an instant-read thermometer inserted into the thickest part of a wing away from bone registers 165°F, about 4½ minutes. Using a slotted spoon, transfer the wings to the prepared plate to drain. Then, transfer to a large platter and sprinkle each wing with an equal amount of the ganja salt. Serve hot.

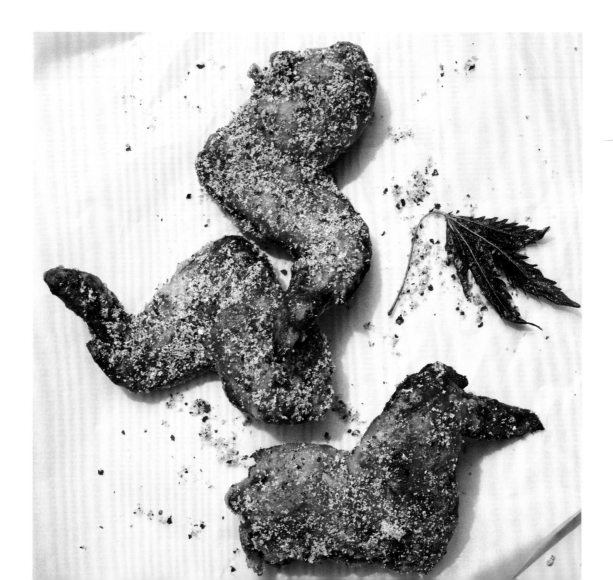

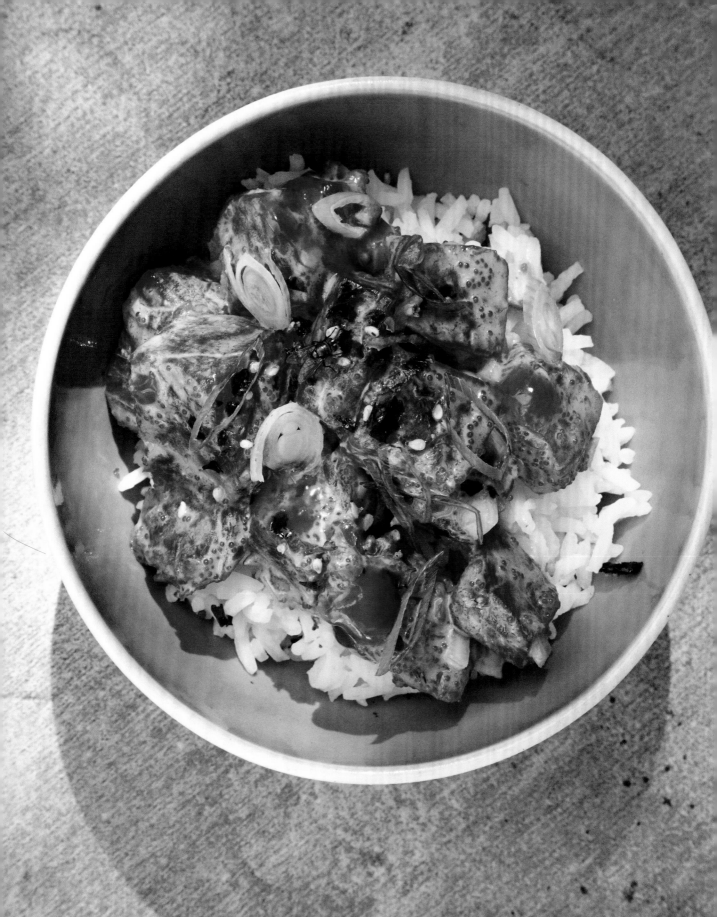

THC

2.3 mg per serving;
18.4 mg total recipe

With kief: 7.8 mg per serving;
62.9 mg total recipe

Pakalolo Poke Bowl

Sheldon Simeon/Tin Roof
Yield: 8 servings

Poke

1 pound sashimi-grade tuna, cut into ½-inch cubes

1 small Vidalia onion, finely chopped

1 teaspoon sea salt

¾-inch piece fresh ginger, peeled and grated

1 tablespoon flower-infused sesame oil (see page 64)

1 tablespoon Sriracha

1 tablespoon sambal oelek

1 tablespoon oyster sauce

2 tablespoons soy sauce

¼ cup masago (capelin roe)

¼ cup mayonnaise

Sweet Soy Sauce

¼ cup soy sauce

¼ cup granulated sugar

1½ tablespoons mirin

1½ tablespoons sake

1 tablespoon Hon Dashi powder (Japanese stock base)

½ cup water, plus 1½ tablespoons

2 tablespoons cornstarch

6 cups cooked long-grain white rice

1 green onion, white and tender green parts, thinly sliced

Furikake (dried Japanese seasoning), Mini Yakko-brand rice crackers, and/or aonori (dried seaweed powder) for garnish

1 gram raw kief (optional)

Chef Sheldon Simeon of Maui's Tin Roof restaurant is a man who takes his poke seriously. When he came through our office to make a traditional poke for us, he casually pulled a dime bag of ground inamona nuts—nearly impossible to find outside of Hawaii, but classic for purists—out of his backpack, knowing that the poke wouldn't be the same without them. Think of weed as the inamona nuts of this less-traditional poke; it just adds that extra something.

To make the poke: In a large bowl, combine the tuna, onion, sea salt, and ginger and fold together to mix evenly. Add the infused sesame oil, Sriracha, sambal oelek, oyster sauce, soy sauce, masago, and mayonnaise and gently fold together until well mixed.

To make the sweet soy sauce: In a small saucepan over medium-high heat, combine the soy sauce, sugar, mirin, sake, dashi powder, and ½ cup water and bring to a boil, stirring occasionally. Lower the heat to a simmer and cook for 10 minutes to blend the flavors.

Meanwhile, in a small bowl, stir together the cornstarch and remaining 1½ tablespoons water to make a slurry. While stirring constantly, slowly add the slurry to the soy sauce mixture, then continue stirring until the mixture thickens to a syrupy consistency. Remove from the heat and set aside to cool.

Divide the rice evenly among eight bowls. Scoop the poke over the rice, dividing it evenly, and drizzle each serving with about 1 tablespoon of the sweet soy sauce. Garnish the rice with the green onion, furikake, and rice crackers, then dust the bowls with the aonori and the kief (if using). Serve immediately.

THC

8.4 mg per serving;
33.4 mg total recipe

Swordfish Teriyaki

Yoya Takahashi/Umi by Hamasaku

Yield: 4 servings

Four 5-ounce swordfish or halibut fillets

Kosher salt and freshly ground black pepper

2 tablespoons flower-infused butter (see page 68)

1½ cups Homemade Teriyaki Sauce (recipe follows)

Toasted sesame seeds for garnish

Green onions, white and tender green parts, sliced, for garnish

Cooked short-grain white rice for serving

So simple, so easy, so good. Frankly, we'd expect nothing less from sushi master Yoya Takahashi of L.A.'s Hamasaku restaurant. Swordfish is a meaty, almost steaky fish, so it does well with strong flavors like this salty-sweet, pot butter–laced teriyaki glaze. Hit this with some toasted sesame seeds and sliced green onions, drop it on a bowl of short-grain rice, and enjoy your night.

Heat the oven to 400°F.

Season the fish all over with salt and pepper.

In a large cast-iron or other heavy ovenproof skillet over medium-high heat, melt the infused butter. When the foam subsides, add the fish and cook until cooked halfway through, about 2½ minutes (timing will depend on the thickness of the fillets; plan on 10 minutes total for fillets 1 inch thick). Flip the fish and transfer the skillet to the oven until the fish is cooked 80 percent through, about 5 minutes.

Return the skillet to the stove top over low heat, pour in the teriyaki sauce, and cook, basting the fish occasionally with the sauce, until the fish is cooked through, about 3 minutes longer. Transfer the fish to a plate and keep warm. Continue reducing the sauce over low heat until thickened, about 10 minutes.

Pour the thickened sauce over the fish, garnish with sesame seeds and green onions, and serve immediately with rice.

Homemade Teriyaki Sauce

Yield: 3½ cups

1 cup mirin	1 cup soy sauce
1 cup sake	½ cup granulated sugar

In a medium bowl, combine the mirin, sake, soy sauce, and sugar and whisk until fully incorporated. Transfer to an airtight container and store in the refrigerator for up to 2 months.

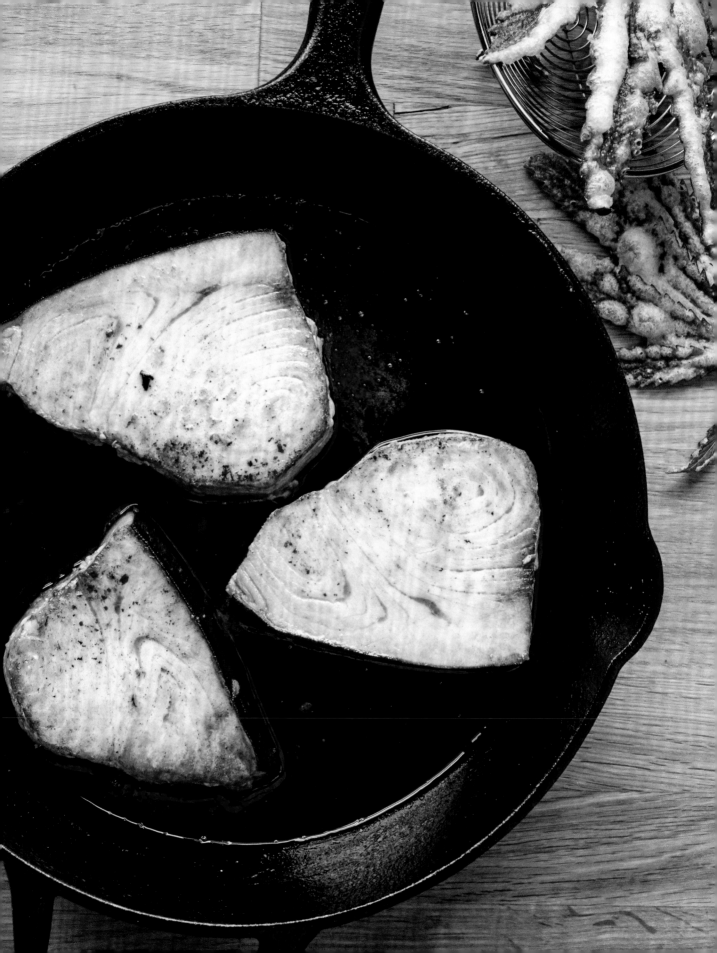

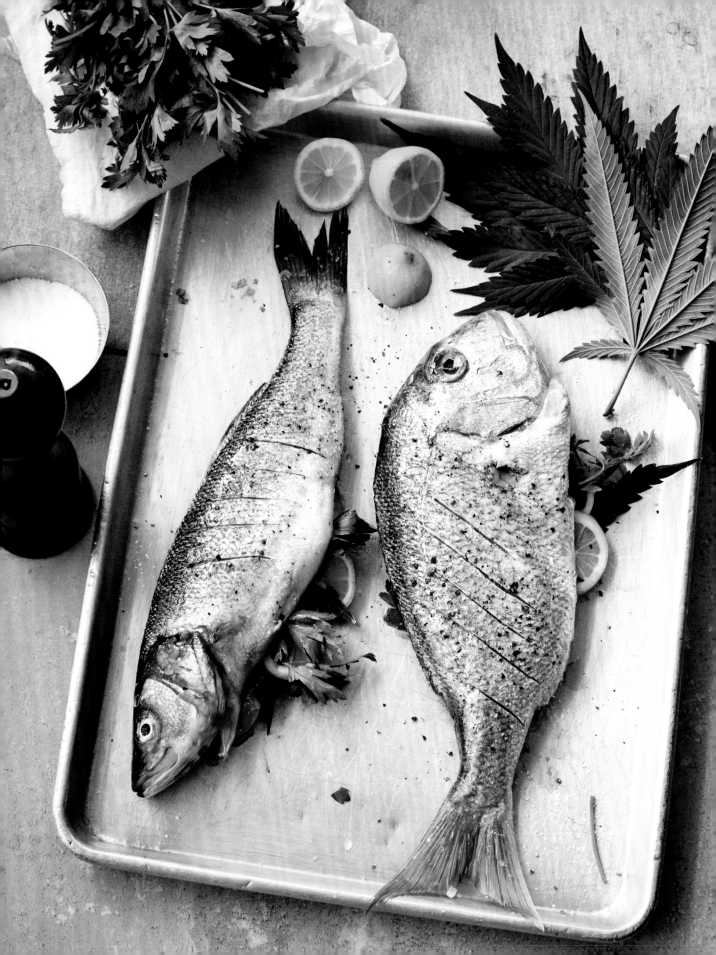

THC

10.4 mg per serving;
41.6 mg total recipe

With rosin and cannabis flower:
38.6 mg per serving;
154.2 mg total recipe

Grilled Whole Sea Bream

David Wilcox/Journeymen

Yield: 4 servings

½ cup flower-infused olive oil
(see page 64)

1 gram rosin (see page 22;
optional)

4 whole, head-on black sea
bream or branzino, cleaned

Kosher salt and freshly ground
black pepper

4 grams cannabis flower, ground
(optional)

3 cups mixed fresh herbs and
greens (such as cannabis fan
leaf, flat-leaf parsley, cilantro,
and miner's lettuce)

2 lemons, thinly sliced, plus
freshly squeezed lemon juice
for dressing

Extra-virgin olive oil for
dressing

Vanessa Says: Fish and cannabis's
bright limonene notes are an ideal
match, especially with the herbs
in this dish. Use a citrus-scented
rosin like Tangie or Lemon Haze
on the inside of the cavity before
stuffing with herbs.

Whole fish stuffed with herbs and grilled over an open fire is a pretty
incredible summer dinner. Grilled whole fish stuffed with herbs *and*
herb—now that's just next-level. When chef David Wilcox of L.A.'s
Journeymen made this on the show, he brushed the fish inside and out
with weed-infused olive oil, then stuffed it with extra rosin and buds.
But Wilcox's specialty is local and foraged ingredients, so he's flexible,
and his recipe is more of a guideline. Pretty much any combination of
herbs, greens, and lettuces will work just fine here, along with as much
rosin and bud as you think your guests may want to handle.

Build a hot fire for direct-heat grilling in a charcoal grill or heat a gas
grill to medium-high.

In a small saucepan over low heat, warm the infused olive oil (just to
the touch). Add the rosin (if using) and stir to dissolve.

Pat the fish dry inside and out. Score the skin in a few places on both
sides of each fish, making the slashes perpendicular to the backbone
and just deep enough to expose some flesh. Rub each fish, inside and
out, with the warm oil, then season liberally inside and out with salt
and pepper. Place 1 gram of the cannabis flower in the cavity of each
fish, then stuff ½ cup of the mixed herbs into each cavity so the cannabis does not fall out. Line each fish cavity with the lemon slices,
overlapping them slightly.

When the fish are ready for grilling, check the heat of the grill; it
is ready when you can hold your hand 5 inches above the heat for
4 to 6 seconds before having to pull it away. Place the fish on the
grill rack and cook for 7 to 9 minutes, flipping them once halfway
through the cooking time. The skin should be crisp and the flesh
supple and opaque throughout.

Just before serving, in a medium bowl, toss the remaining 1 cup
mixed herbs and greens with a splash each of lemon juice and extra-
virgin olive oil and season with salt. Transfer the fish to individual
plates and serve with the dressed greens.

THC

8.4 mg per serving;
50 mg total recipe

Grilled Oysters

MUNCHIES Test Kitchen

Yield: 6 servings

2 tablespoons olive oil

1 bunch ramps, trimmed and
thinly sliced

¾ cup plus 2 tablespoons
unsalted butter, at room
temperature, plus more for
the coals

3 tablespoons flower-infused
butter (see page 68)

Grated zest and juice of 1 lemon

Kosher salt and freshly ground
black pepper

36 oysters

There are basically two truths about oysters: They are a great way to start off a meal, and they are a total pain in the ass to shuck, especially for a crowd. Make someone else shuck the oysters while you set up the grill. You'll hear some complaining, but that will stop when the weed butter hits. If you can't find ramps at your local store or don't know where to forage for them in the wild, substitute the tops of green or spring onions and a garlic clove or two.

In a 10-inch skillet over medium-high heat, warm the olive oil. Add the ramps and cook, stirring often, until soft, 2 to 3 minutes. Transfer to a bowl; add both butters, the lemon zest, and lemon juice; and mix well. Season with salt and pepper and then set aside.

Using an oyster knife, shuck each oyster, lifting off and discarding the top shell and leaving the oyster in the bottom (more cup-shaped) shell. Slide the knife under the oyster to sever the muscle attaching it to the shell.

Light a fire for direct-heat grilling in a charcoal grill. Once hot, place a small dollop of unsalted butter directly on the coals and cover the grill until it starts to smoke.

Top each oyster with an equal amount of the butter mixture. Place the oysters on the grill rack and immediately cover the grill. Cook until the oysters are plump and their edges begin to curl slightly, 2 to 3 minutes. Using tongs, carefully transfer the oysters to individual plates or a couple of large serving platters. Serve immediately.

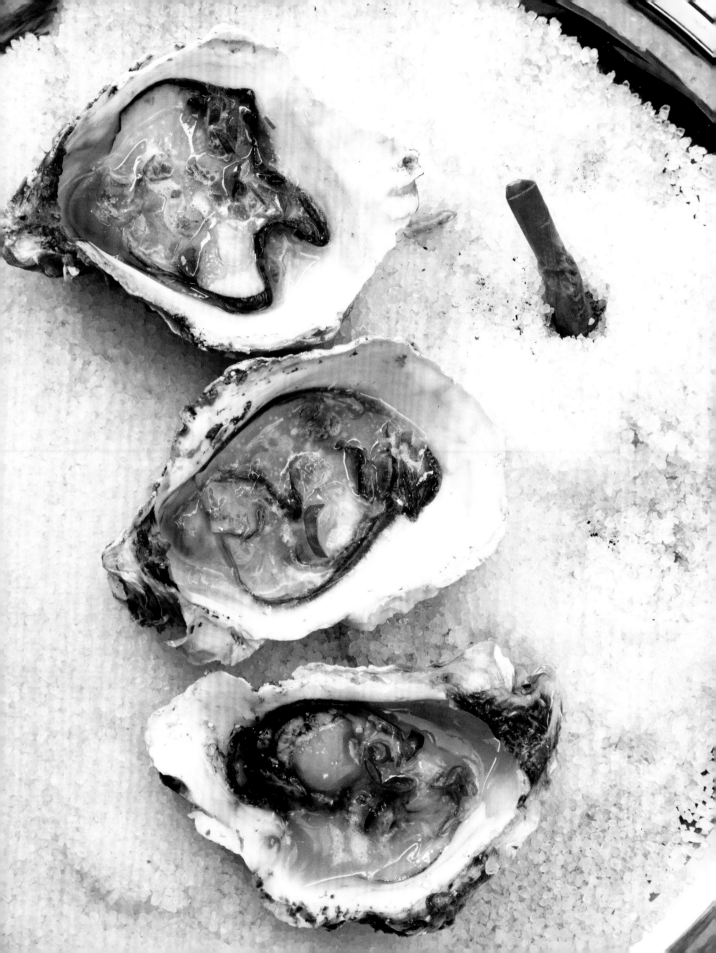

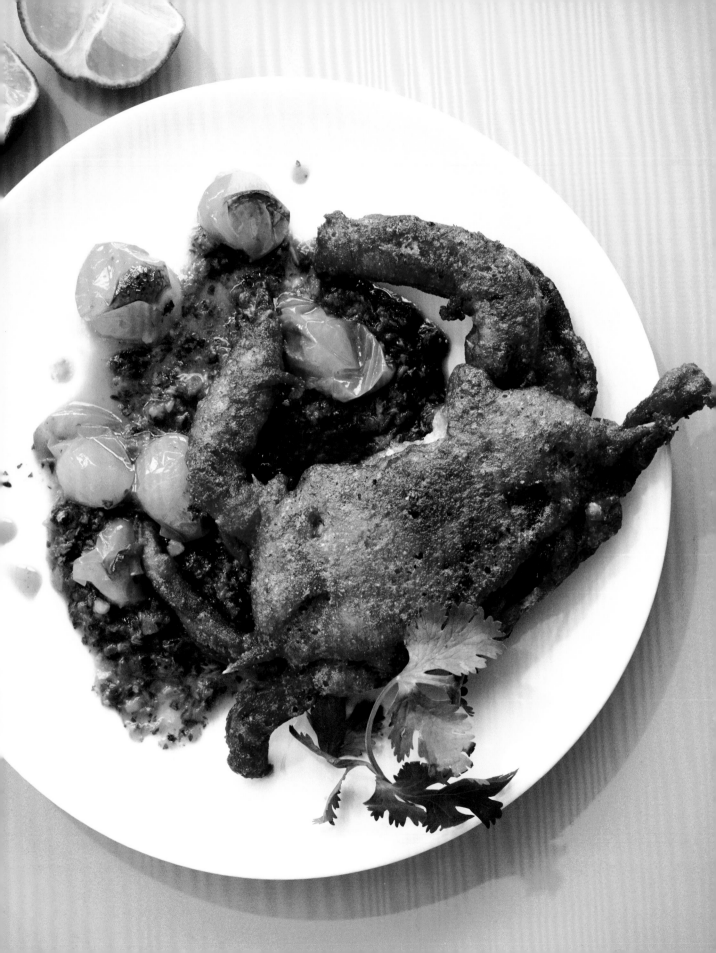

THC
5.2 mg per serving;
41.6 mg total recipe

Fried Soft–Shell Crab with Shishito Pepper Mole

Daniela Soto-Innes/Cosme/Atla
Yield: 8 servings

Mole

¼ cup flower-infused olive oil (see page 64)

¼ cup olive oil

3 garlic cloves, sliced

7 ounces shishito peppers, stemmed

8 serrano chiles, halved and seeded

Leaves and tender stems from 1 bunch cilantro

1 cup small ice cubes

1 tablespoon kosher salt

3 tablespoons yuzu juice

3 tablespoons freshly squeezed lime juice

Tempura Batter

1½ cups cornstarch

1 cup corn flour

1 tablespoon baking soda

1 teaspoon kosher salt

2 cups soda water, chilled

1½ cups cornstarch

Vegetable oil for frying

8 soft-shell crabs, cleaned (your fishmonger can do this for you)

Soft-shell crabs done right don't actually need much in the way of accompaniments, but this recipe, from Daniela Soto-Innes of New York City's Mexican legend Cosme and all-day cafe Atla, blew our fucking minds. Perfectly crunchy, juicy fried soft-shell crabs might not *need* a just-spicy enough (and just-heady enough) shishito pepper mole and smoky roasted tomatoes, but you'll never want to eat them without either again. Plus, adding the infused oil to the mole makes portioning and dosing this dish easy. The combination of cornstarch and corn flour keeps the crabs crunchy; look for corn flour in well-stocked supermarkets, natural food stores, or online.

To make the mole: In a medium saucepan over medium heat, warm both oils. When the combined oil is hot, add the garlic and cook, stirring, until translucent, about 1 minute. Add the shishitos and serranos and cook, stirring occasionally, until the shishitos burst, about 5 minutes. Transfer the contents of the pan to a blender. Add the cilantro, ice cubes, salt, yuzu juice, and lime juice and process until smooth. Pass through a fine-mesh strainer into a medium bowl and set aside at room temperature.

To make the tempura batter: In a medium bowl, stir together the cornstarch, corn flour, baking soda, and salt. Transfer to the freezer and chill for 20 minutes. Remove from the freezer and stir in the soda water; the batter should be relatively thick. Keep the batter refrigerated until ready to use.

Line a baking sheet with paper towels and set near the stove. Spread the 1½ cups cornstarch in a wide, shallow medium bowl.

Pour the vegetable oil to a depth of 2 inches in a heavy, medium stockpot and heat to 375°F on a deep-frying (candy) thermometer. Working with one crab at a time, dredge the crab in the cornstarch,

continued

Fried Soft-Shell Crab with Shishito Pepper Mole, *continued*

Roasted Tomatoes

1 pint yellow cherry tomatoes

2 tablespoons olive oil

1 teaspoon kosher salt

8 limes, halved

40 fresh lemon balm leaves

Vanessa Says: When I see cilantro, I think of the cannabis fan leaves. More tender, smaller leaves blitzed with the tender cilantro leaves will add another depth to this mole. The shiso flavor of the leaves will play off the yuzu acid notes.

coating evenly on all sides and tapping off the excess. Using tongs, dip the crab into the batter, letting the excess drip off, then lower the crab gently into the hot oil. Fry until golden and crispy, turning it once at the halfway point, 4 minutes total. Using the tongs, transfer the crab to the prepared baking sheet to drain.

To make the roasted tomatoes: Heat the broiler. Line a baking sheet with parchment paper.

Pile the tomatoes on the prepared baking sheet. Drizzle with the olive oil, sprinkle with the salt, and toss to coat evenly. Spread the tomatoes in a single layer and broil just until they begin to burst, 2 to 3 minutes.

Divide the mole evenly among individual plates, spreading it out, and top each plate with a few tomatoes and a crab. Squeeze a lime half over each crab and garnish with 5 lemon balm leaves. Alternatively, spread the mole on a large serving platter, top with the tomatoes and crabs, squeeze half of the lime halves over the top, and garnish with the lemon balm leaves. Serve immediately, with the remaining lime halves on the side.

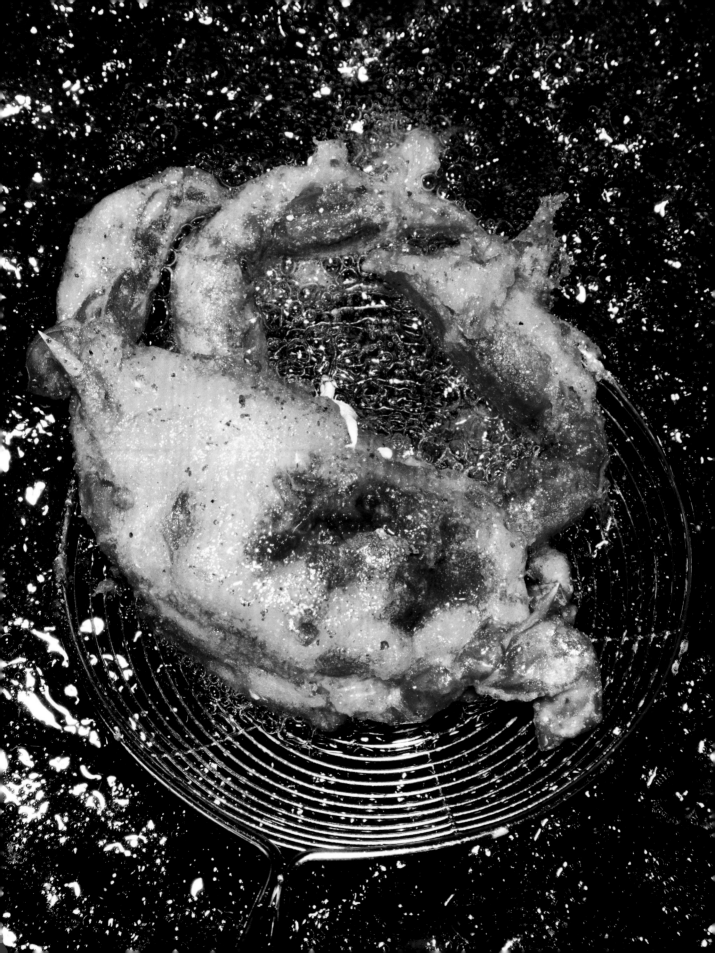

THC
3.3 mg per serving;
20 mg total recipe

Green Shellfish Curry

Louis Tikaram/E.P & L.P.

Yield: 6 servings

4 cups chicken stock

1 cup coconut cream

¼ cup makrut lime leaves

2 lemongrass stalks, grass tops removed and then bashed to release flavor

¼ cup Homemade Curry Paste (facing page)

2 tablespoons fish sauce, plus more as needed

2 tablespoons oyster sauce

1 tablespoon granulated sugar, plus more as needed

1 pound sea scallops

1 pound mussels, scrubbed and debearded

½ cup firmly packed fresh Thai basil leaves

2 Fresno chiles, seeded and cut lengthwise into narrow strips

2 Thai eggplants, quartered through the stem end

2 tablespoons tamarind liquid (see Note)

Steamed jasmine rice for serving

Louis Tikaram, chef at E.P & L.P. in Los Angeles, puts the "green" in green curry with this seafood-packed, wildly flavorful Thai coconut stew. When Tikaram came through the *Bong Appétit* house, he added weed in six different forms (high-cannabinoid full-spectrum extract, kief, flower rosin, CBD crystalline, THCA crystalline, and fire OG flower, if you're keeping track) to make this curry pack a powerful punch, but this version doesn't require you to live *that* large. This recipe makes more curry paste than you need; freeze the extra in an ice-cube tray so you're never that far from green curry bliss.

In a medium saucepan over high heat, combine the chicken stock, coconut cream, lime leaves, and lemongrass and bring to a boil. Lower the heat to a simmer, stir in the curry paste, and let simmer for 5 minutes to blend the flavors. Add the fish sauce, oyster sauce, and sugar and stir to mix.

Add the scallops and mussels (discarding any mussels that fail to close to the touch) to the pan and cook at a gentle simmer until the mussels have begun to open and the scallops are partially cooked but still translucent at the center, about 3 minutes. Stir in the basil, chiles, and eggplants and continue to simmer until the scallops are opaque throughout and all of the mussels are open (discard any that failed to open), about 3 minutes longer. The vegetables should still be nice and firm.

Stir in the tamarind liquid and adjust the seasoning with more sugar or fish sauce, if needed. Serve hot with the rice.

Note: To make tamarind liquid, in a small bowl, soak about 3 tablespoons tamarind pulp (sold in small, cellophane-wrapped blocks in Asian stores) in ½ cup warm water for about 15 minutes, pressing against and squeezing the pulp every now and again to soften it. Then, pour the contents of the bowl through a fine-mesh strainer placed over a second bowl and press against the solids in the strainer to force through as much of the thin puree as possible. Discard the solids. Measure what you need for the curry, then store the remainder in a tightly sealed jar in the refrigerator for up to 1 week.

THC
20 mg per ¼ cup;
240 mg total recipe

Homemade Curry Paste

Yield: 3 cups

1½ cups long, red dried chiles, seeded

1 cup peeled and sliced galangal

3 lemongrass stalks; grassy tops, tough outer leaves, and base removed; thinly sliced

½ cup peeled and sliced turmeric root

½ cup garlic cloves

½ cup sliced wild ginger (karachi)

1 tablespoon shrimp paste

3 grams cannabis flower, ground and decarboxylated (see page 55)

In a medium bowl, combine the chiles with warm water to cover and let soak for 20 minutes. Drain, discarding the liquid, and transfer the chiles to a blender or food processor. Add the galangal, lemongrass, turmeric root, garlic, ginger, shrimp paste, and cannabis flower and process until smooth, adding a little water if needed for the blades to move freely. Transfer to an airtight container and store in the refrigerator for up to 1 week or in the freezer for up to 1 month.

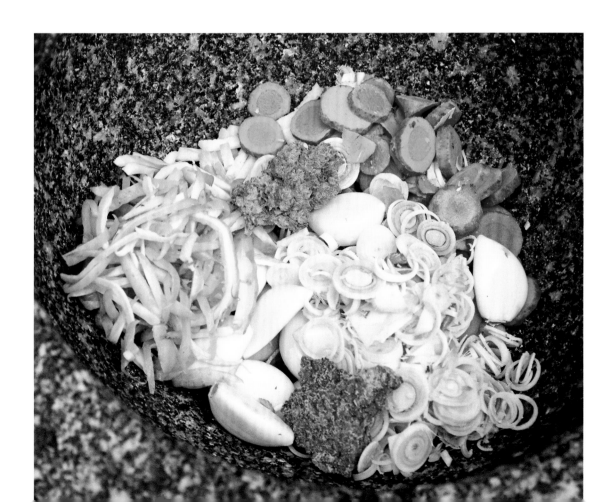

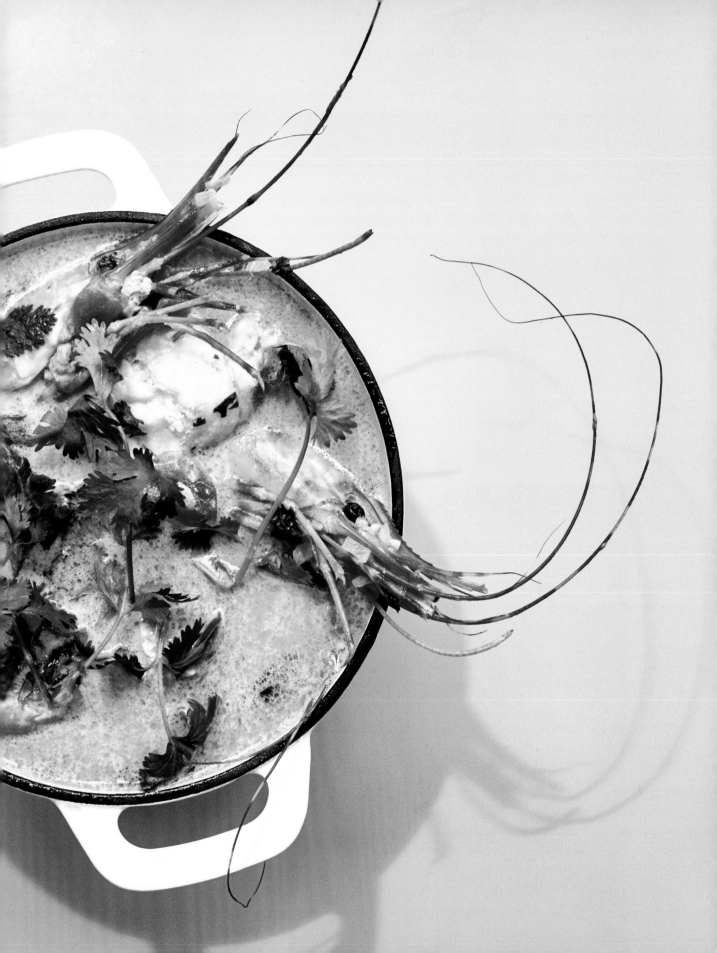

THC

11.7 mg per serving;
93.6 mg total recipe

With live resin:
33.7 mg per serving;
293.6 mg total recipe

Coconut Seafood Stew (Moqueca)

Natalia Pereira/Woodspoon

Yield: 8 servings

3 pounds skinned black cod fillet, cut into 2-inch pieces

½ cup olive oil

4 tablespoons freshly squeezed lime juice

3 garlic cloves, minced

Leaves and tender stems of 1 bunch cilantro, coarsely chopped

2 yellow onions, finely chopped

1 cup weed-infused coconut milk (see page 71)

2 cups coconut milk

3 tablespoons palm oil

6 tomatoes, chopped

1 pound large head-on prawns

1 tablespoon kosher salt

This ultra-comforting Brazilian seafood stew from chef Natalia Pereira of L.A.'s Woodspoon is called *moqueca*. Its long-simmered flavor completely belies the fact that it cooks for only 20 minutes and that the hardest thing you have to do here is infuse coconut milk. Palm oil is traditional, and there isn't really a substitute; but if you can't find it, use any neutral oil instead.

In a large bowl, toss the cod with 3 tablespoons of the olive oil, 2 tablespoons of the lime juice, one-third of the garlic, and half of the cilantro. Let sit for 10 minutes.

Meanwhile, in a large saucepan over medium-high, warm the remaining 5 tablespoons olive oil. Add the remaining garlic and the onions and cook, stirring often, until the onions are soft, about 4 minutes. Stir in both coconut milks, the palm oil, and tomatoes and bring to a boil. Lower the heat to a simmer and stir in the cod and prawns. Cook until the cod is opaque throughout and the prawns have turned pink, about 8 minutes. Season with the salt, stir in the remaining cilantro, and serve immediately.

Vanessa Says: Coconut milk has a healthy amount of fat that is great for holding THC and flavor. At the end of the infusion, add 0.25 gram live resin to the coconut milk. Fragrant with delicate terpenes, the stew will take on a new dimension.

THC
18 mg per serving;
108 mg total recipe

Confit Octopus

MUNCHIES Test Kitchen

Yield: 6 servings

One 4-pound octopus, cleaned
(ask your fishmonger do this
for you)

Kosher salt

2 garlic cloves, smashed

1 bunch oregano, plus
2 tablespoons oregano leaves

½ cup canola oil

2 cups olive oil

4 tablespoons flower-infused
olive oil (see page 64)

3 tablespoons red wine vinegar

15 Castelvetrano olives, pitted
and lightly crushed

3 celery stalks, thinly sliced
on the diagonal

1 small red onion, thinly sliced

One 15-ounce can chickpeas,
drained and rinsed

Freshly ground black pepper

We know octopus can look a little intimidating, even if you're *not* high.
All those tentacles. All those suction cups. But octopus has a secret:
it's actually wildly easy to cook. You put it in some liquid, let it cook
low and slow, forget about it for a while, and then you come back and
it's perfect. MUNCHIES' own Action Bronson is a big fan of dabbing
while waiting for his octopus to be done, but since you're poaching
this guy in infused olive oil, you don't even need to. But that's not to
say you can't. We're not going to tell you how to live your life.

Season the octopus tentacles with salt and place in a large saucepan
along with the garlic, oregano bunch, canola oil, regular olive oil,
and 2 tablespoons of the infused olive oil. Bring to a low simmer,
uncovered, over medium heat and cook until tender, about 1 hour.
The octopus is ready when a knife tip slides easily into the thickest part of a tentacle. Using tongs, transfer the octopus to a cutting
board, let cool until it can be handled, then cut the tentacles on
the diagonal into ½-inch pieces and transfer to a bowl.

Let the tentacles cool to room temperature. Add the remaining
2 tablespoons infused oil, vinegar, olives, celery, onion, and chickpeas and toss to mix. Season with salt and pepper, add the oregano
leaves, and toss again. Transfer to a platter and serve immediately.

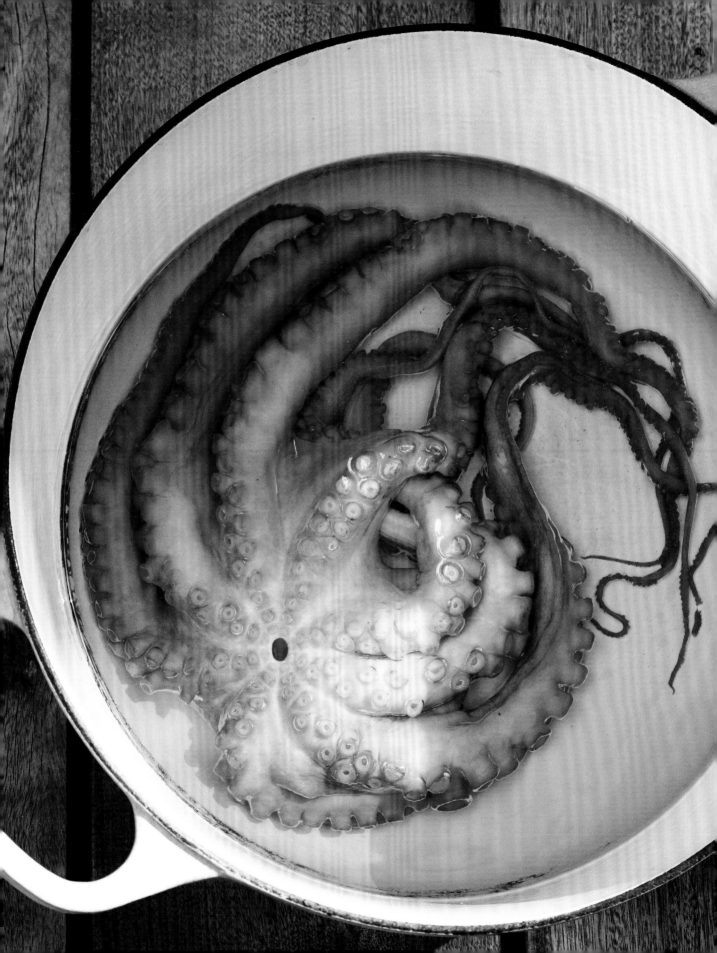

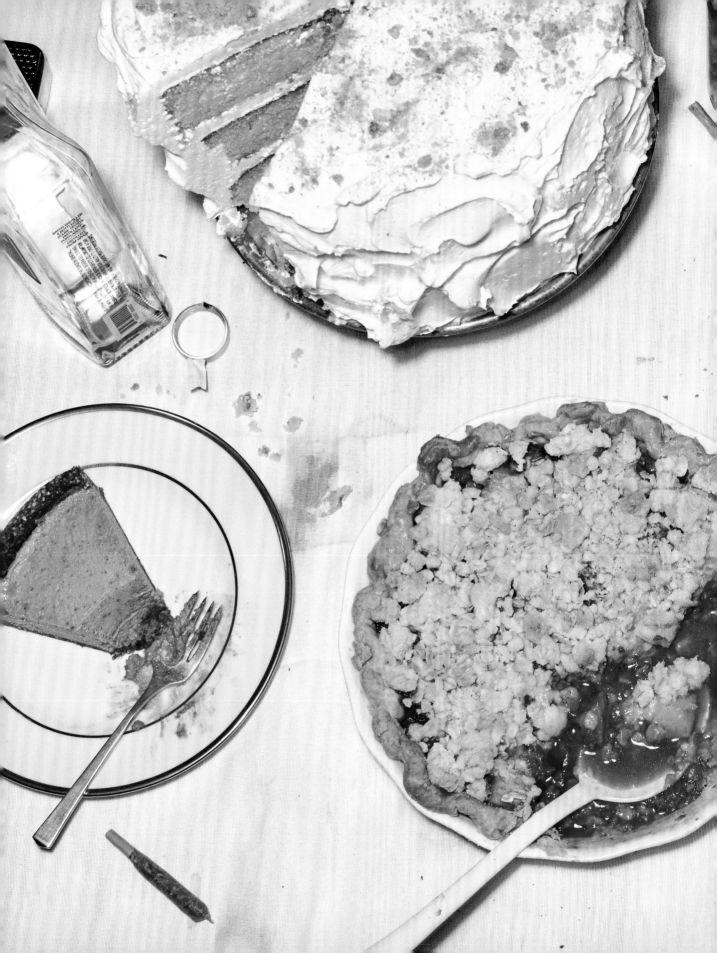

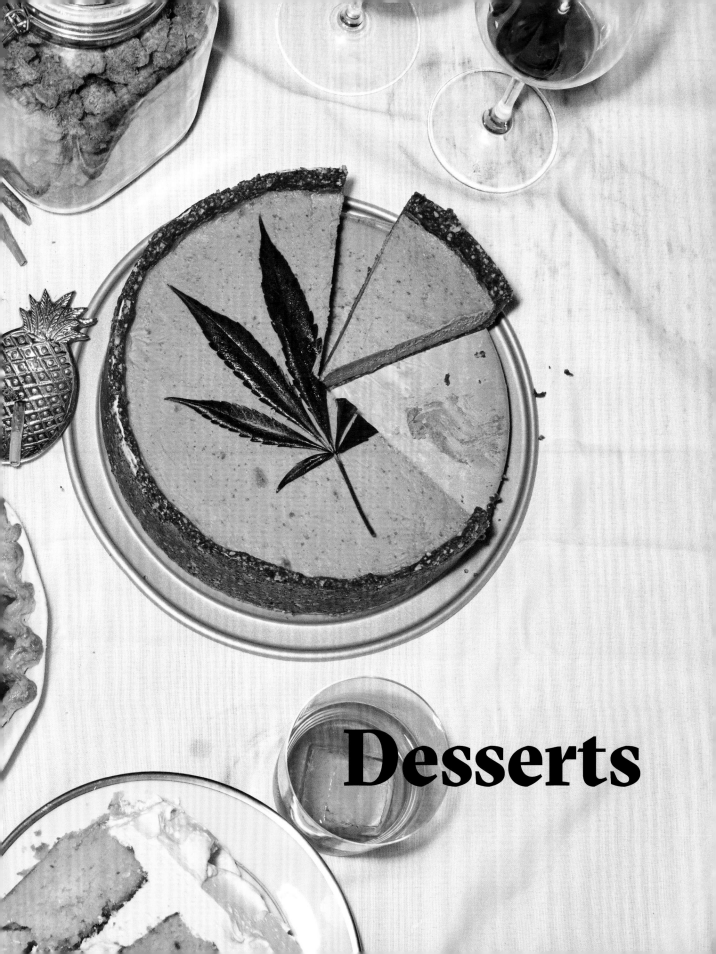

Desserts

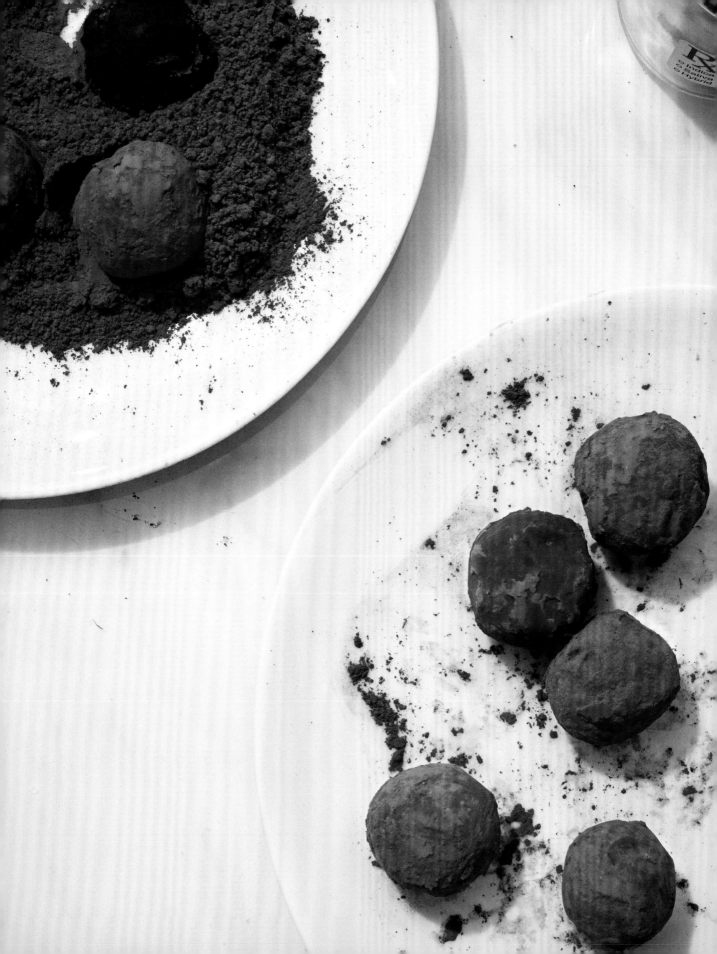

THC
5 mg per truffle;
160 mg total recipe

Truffles

Vanessa Lavorato

Yield: 32 truffles

1 cup finely chopped
good-quality dark chocolate
(66% cacao)

5 tablespoons weed-infused
cream (see page 72)

3 tablespoons heavy cream

1 tablespoon bourbon

1 tablespoon honey

1 pinch kosher salt

1 tablespoon unsalted butter,
at room temperature

⅛ teaspoon vanilla extract

1 cup cocoa powder

Imagine how sick it would be to show up to someone's party with a box of these. "Oh, it's nothing. Just a box of bud-and-bourbon-infused chocolate truffles I made myself." You'd be invited literally everywhere after that. Bourbon is Vanessa's all-time favorite alcohol in the kitchen. Use a good bourbon and a dark chocolate here. The honey complements the liquor and adds a nice shine to the ganache. These truffles make the perfect host gift that is sure to be the highlight of the night. Vanessa microdoses them for a reason, *non c'è due senza tre* is italian for "betcha can't eat just one."

Place the chocolate in a small metal bowl.

In a small saucepan over medium heat, combine both creams, the bourbon, honey, and salt. Cook, stirring constantly, until the cream just starts to bubble. Pour the warm cream over the chocolate and let sit for 5 minutes.

Using a rubber spatula, stir the mixture slowly, working in small circles from the center and moving outward until all the ingredients are incorporated and the chocolate has melted. Once the mixture reaches 95°F on an instant-read thermometer, add the butter and vanilla and stir well to combine. Refrigerate the ganache for about 2 hours, until firm.

Place the cocoa powder in a large bowl.

Roll, scoop, or pipe the ganache into 1-teaspoon balls. Toss the balls in the cocoa powder to coat completely. Transfer to an airtight container and store in the refrigerator for up to 1 week.

THC
1.1 mg per piece;
66.8 mg total recipe

Stoner Candy Bites

Thu Tran

Yield: 60 pieces

2 cups crushed potato chips
(we recommend Kettle brand
with sea salt)

2 cups crushed thin pretzels

2 cups crushed corn flakes or
Corn Chex

4 tablespoons flower-infused
butter (see page 68)

2 cups mini marshmallows

4 cups semisweet
chocolate chips

½ pound unsweetened
chocolate, coarsely chopped

4 tablespoons candy sprinkles
(optional)

Maldon sea salt (optional)

Vanessa Says: Add a tablespoon of
infused coconut oil to the chocolate.
It will make the chocolate thinner
and easier to work with as well as
up the dose.

Thu Tran is the delightful creative genius behind *Food Party*, a show that
blends cooking with puppets, interactive snacks, and pure unadulter-
ated weirdness. It's an amazing thing to watch when you're high. And
since you're already high, you may as well be eating this candy, the
finest stoner snack known to man—sweet, salty, chocolaty, crunchy,
and chewy, all in one tiny package.

Line a 9 by 13-inch sheet pan with parchment paper and set aside. In
a large bowl, combine the potato chips, pretzels, and corn flakes and
set aside.

In a medium saucepan over medium heat, melt the infused butter.
Add the marshmallows and cook, stirring, until melted and smooth,
about 5 minutes. Pour the marshmallow-butter mixture over the
potato chips mixture and stir to mix well. Transfer the mixture to
the prepared sheet pan and spread in an even layer, pressing it to
flatten. Refrigerate for about 30 minutes, until cool.

Pour water to a depth of 2 inches in a medium saucepan and bring to a
gentle simmer over low heat. Put the chocolate chips and unsweetened
chocolate in a heatproof bowl and set the bowl over (not touching) the
water in the saucepan. Heat, stirring, until chocolate has melted and
is smooth.

Spread the warm chocolate over the mixture in the pan. Top with the
sprinkles or a scattering of sea salt, if desired. Refrigerate, uncovered,
until cooled completely. Cut the potato chip–marshmallow mixture
into sixty 2 by 1-inch pieces. Transfer to an airtight container and
store in the refrigerator for up to 5 days.

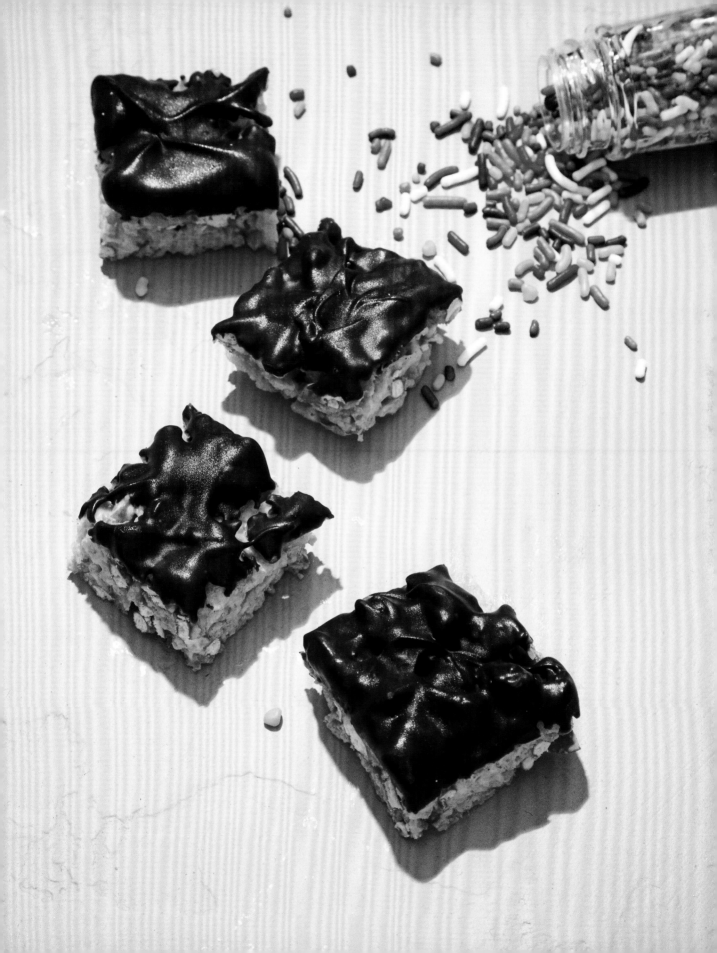

THC
6 mg per ice pop;
66.8 mg total recipe

With infused cream:
18 mg per ice pop;
200.6 mg total recipe

Frozen Cocoa Pudding Pops

Kelly Fields/Willa Jean
Yield: 11 ice pops

1¼ cups heavy cream, plus
¼ cup regular or weed-infused
cream (see page 72)

1½ cups whole milk

½ vanilla bean, split lengthwise

½ cup granulated sugar

2 tablespoons cocoa powder

Kosher salt

2 large eggs

4 tablespoons flower-infused
butter (see page 68), at room
temperature, cubed

¼ pound bittersweet chocolate
(70% cacao; we recommend
Valrhona brand), coarsely
chopped

Kelly Fields, chef and partner at Willa Jean in New Orleans, may or may not be the person who invented frozen rosé—the history is hazy, and there are a lot of pretenders to the throne; for the record, we believe her. But she's definitely the person who came up with the equally brilliant idea of putting drugs in Fudgsicles. If you don't have ice-pop molds, you can just freeze the base in a plastic container and scoop it like ice cream, keeping in mind that the dosage will change depending on the size of the scoops.

In a medium, heavy saucepan over medium-high heat, combine the heavy cream, milk, and vanilla bean and warm just to scalding (tiny bubbles begin to form along the sides of the pan).

Meanwhile, in a medium bowl, whisk together the sugar, cocoa powder, and 2 teaspoons salt. Add the eggs and whisk until smooth.

When the cream-milk mixture is ready, remove it from the heat. Add about ¼ cup of the hot liquid to the egg-sugar mixture while whisking constantly. Continue whisking in the hot liquid, ¼ cup at a time, until most of the hot liquid is incorporated into the egg mixture. Then whisk the cream-egg mixture into cream mixture remaining in the saucepan and place over medium heat. Cook, whisking constantly, until the mixture thickens and bubbles, about 5 minutes. Remove from the heat and immediately whisk in the infused butter and chocolate until melted.

Remove and discard the vanilla bean. Taste and adjust with salt, if needed. Let cool slightly, portion into 3-ounce ice-pop molds, and freeze until set. Store in the freezer for up to 1 month.

THC

14.8 mg per serving;
133.8 mg total recipe

With whipped weed-infused
honey: 18.8 mg per serving;
171.2 mg total recipe

Honey Rosemary Ice Cream

Mindy Segal

Yield: nine ½-cup servings

2 cups whole milk

1¾ cups heavy cream

¼ cup weed-infused cream
(see page 72)

4 rosemary sprigs, stems
removed and reserved and
leaves coarsely chopped

1 cup granulated sugar

13 egg yolks

½ cup whipped weed-infused
honey (see page 74; optional)

1 teaspoon vanilla extract

½ teaspoon kosher salt

Mindy Segal is a pastry chef and cookie genius who was among the first serious chefs to get into commercial edibles. She's elevated the use of cannabis in sweets to an art form, an accomplishment that's clear on first taste of this herby-sweet ice cream. Use a strain high in pinene, like Northern Lights, in your infused cream to play up the rosemary, or swap in some whipped infused honey to play up the get-you-baked-ness.

In a medium saucepan over medium-low heat, combine the milk, both creams, and rosemary leaves and stems and warm for 1 hour. Take care the mixture does not boil or scald. You are simply infusing over low heat at this stage.

Meanwhile, in a large bowl, whisk the sugar and egg yolks until blended. When the cream mixture is ready, bring it just to a boil, remove from the heat, and slowly pour it into yolk mixture while whisking constantly until fully combined. Pour the mixture back into the saucepan and cook over medium heat, stirring constantly, until thick, about 25 minutes.

Remove the pan from the heat and stir in the honey (if using), vanilla, and salt. Let cool for several minutes, then cover and refrigerate until cold.

Strain the mixture through a fine-mesh strainer set over a bowl. Transfer to an ice-cream maker and freeze according to the manufacturer's instructions. Scoop into an airtight container, transfer to the freezer, and store for up to 1 month.

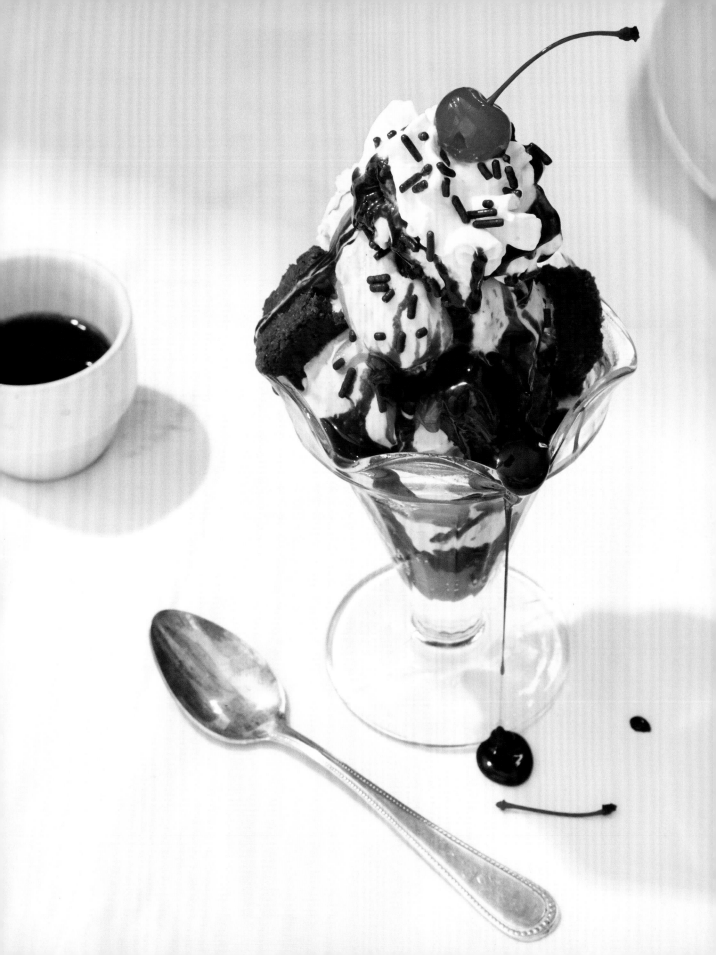

THC

5.5 mg per brownie;
66.8 mg total recipe

With infused peanut butter
sauce and infused whipped
cream: 26.2 mg per serving;
310.6 mg total recipe

Brownies

6 tablespoons flower-infused
butter (see page 68)

4 tablespoons unsalted butter

¼ pound bittersweet chocolate
(70% cacao; we recommend
Valrhona brand), coarsely
chopped

¼ pound semisweet chocolate,
coarsely chopped

2 large eggs

1 cup granulated sugar

2 teaspoons vanilla extract

¼ teaspoon kosher salt

1 cup cake flour, sifted

Peanut Butter Sauce

1½ cups Homemade
Peanut Butter (page 232)

2 cups granulated sugar

1 cup water

Vanilla ice cream for serving

Whipped Weed-Infused Cream
(page 73) for serving

Chocolate sauce for serving

Candy sprinkles for serving

Maraschino cherries for serving

Vanessa Says: Infuse the whipped
cream with a fragrant variety like
Forbidden Fruit for a THC cherry
on top of your sundae.

Brownie Sundae

MUNCHIES Test Kitchen
Yield: 12 sundaes

At this point, is there a single recipe more clichéd than the pot brownie? But it seemed wrong not to include one. Eat it as is and revel in your basicness, or put it in a sundae with ice cream, weed-laced peanut butter sauce, chocolate sauce, whipped infused cream, sprinkles, and a cherry— because you're worth it.

To make the brownies: Heat the oven to 400°F. Grease a 9 by 13-inch baking pan, line with parchment paper, and then grease the parchment. Set aside.

Pour water to a depth of 2 inches in a medium saucepan and bring to a simmer. Put both butters and both chocolates in a heatproof bowl and set the bowl over (not touching) the water in the saucepan. Heat, stirring, until the mixture is melted and smooth, about 5 minutes. Remove from the heat and set aside.

In a medium bowl, whisk the eggs until blended. Add the sugar, vanilla, and salt and whisk until incorporated. Stir in the chocolate mixture, mixing well, and then fold in the flour until no white streaks remain. Transfer to the prepared pan, spreading evenly.

Bake until a thin skin forms on top and a toothpick inserted into the center comes out with a few moist crumbs clinging to it, 18 to 20 minutes. Transfer the pan to a wire rack and let cool completely. Cut into twelve 3 by 4-inch brownies. Transfer to an airtight container and store at room temperature for up to 5 days.

To make the peanut butter sauce: In a small saucepan over medium-low heat, combine the peanut butter, sugar, and water and cook, stirring, until the peanut butter and sugar melt and the sauce is smooth, about 5 minutes. Remove from the heat and let cool. Transfer to an airtight container and store in the refrigerator for up to 1 week. Reheat gently before serving.

For each serving, place a brownie in a bowl or parfait glass. Top with a scoop of ice cream, a heaping 1 tablespoon whipped cream, 3 tablespoons of the peanut butter sauce, as much chocolate sauce as you like, a scattering of sprinkles, and a cherry.

THC
3.7 mg per cookie;
66.8 mg total recipe

Salted Chocolate Chip Cookies

MUNCHIES Test Kitchen

Yield: 18 cookies

1¾ cups all-purpose flour

¾ teaspoon baking soda

½ teaspoon kosher salt

4 tablespoons flower-infused
butter (see page 68),
at room temperature

4 tablespoons unsalted butter,
at room temperature

2 tablespoons granulated sugar

1 cup firmly packed light
brown sugar

1 large egg

½ vanilla bean, split lengthwise

½ pound semisweet chocolate,
coarsely chopped

Maldon sea salt

Vanessa Says: You can also swap a
store-bought infused chocolate bar
for the chocolate in this recipe. Chop
it up, keeping in mind the milligrams, to get you to the right dose.

Everyone needs one perfect chocolate chip cookie recipe in their
arsenal, and it may as well be one that gets you blazed. Chopping the
chocolate into irregular chunks (use a serrated knife for that) ensures
there's a bit of chocolate in every bite.

Line two baking sheets with parchment paper. Set aside.

In a medium bowl, stir together the flour, baking soda, and kosher
salt. In a large bowl, combine both butters and beat with a wooden
spoon until soft and smooth. Add both sugars to the butter and
beat until the mixture is lighter in color and fluffy. Add the egg
and beat until incorporated. Using the tip of a knife, scrape the
seeds from the vanilla bean, add to the bowl, and stir to mix well.
Add the flour mixture and stir just until full incorporated, then
fold in the chocolate.

Divide the dough into eighteen equal portions, shape each portion
into a ball, and arrange the balls on the prepared baking sheets,
spacing them about 2 inches apart. Sprinkle each ball with a healthy
pinch of Maldon salt, then refrigerate, uncovered, for 2 hours.

Heat the oven to 375°F.

Bake the cookies, directly from the refrigerator, until set on the
outside but still soft in the middle, about 10 minutes. Remove from
the oven and transfer the cookies to a wire rack to cool slightly.
Transfer to an airtight container and store at room temperature
for up to 1 week.

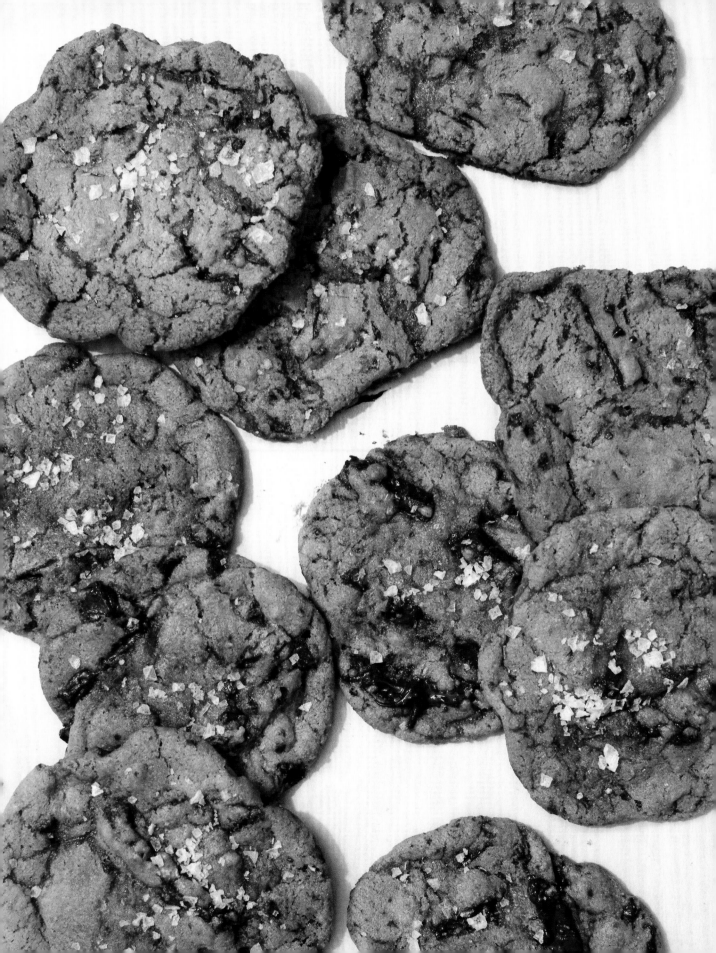

THC
8.4 mg per slice;
66.8 mg total recipe

Raspberry and Peach Pie

Tracy Obolsky/Rockaway Beach Bakery
Yield: 8 equal slices

Pie Crust

3¼ cups plus 2 tablespoons cake flour

3½ teaspoons granulated sugar

¾ teaspoon kosher salt

½ cup cold flower-infused butter (see page 68), cubed

½ cup cold unsalted butter, cubed

¼ cup shortening, frozen and cut into chunks

½ cup plus 3 tablespoons ice-cold water

1 large egg, plus 1 egg yolk

Oat Crumble

½ cup plus 1 tablespoon unsalted butter

½ teaspoon vanilla extract

1¼ cups all-purpose flour

1 cup old-fashioned rolled oats

1 cup granulated sugar

½ teaspoon kosher salt

Tracy Obolsky runs New York's Rockaway Beach Bakery, a sick bakery out in Queens where she's basically the queen of putting butter in things (her croissant game is top-notch). So it's not shocking that her pie crust is impeccable—whether it involves infused butter or not. This pie showcases her skills on all counts: juicy filling, tender oat-crumble topping, and a flaky, shattery crust that also gets you high. Just remember that half of the dough is being saved for a second pie crust; so if you use it all for a double-crust pie, the total THC would be about 133.6 mg.

To make the pie crust: In a large bowl, stir together the flour, granulated sugar, and salt. Scatter both butters over the top and, using your fingers, mix the butters with the flour until pea-size crumbles form. Add the shortening and mix again to form small crumbles. Drizzle the water over the flour mixture, lifting and turning the mixture as you go so the water is evenly distributed and a shaggy dough begins to form. Do not overmix. Press the dough into a rough mass, then divide it in half. You will need only half of the dough for this recipe. Flatten each half into a disk about 1 inch thick. Wrap one disk in plastic wrap and refrigerate for 1 hour to use for this pie. Double wrap the remaining disk and freeze for up to 1 month; thaw overnight in the refrigerator before using.

Grease a 9-inch pie plate.

On a lightly floured surface, roll out the dough into a 12-inch round. Transfer the dough round to the prepared pie plate, pressing it gently onto the bottom and sides. Trim away the excess dough, leaving a roughly ¾-inch overhang. Turn the overhang under itself and then flute the edge or press the edge with floured fork tines. Refrigerate for 30 minutes.

Heat the oven to 350°F.

continued

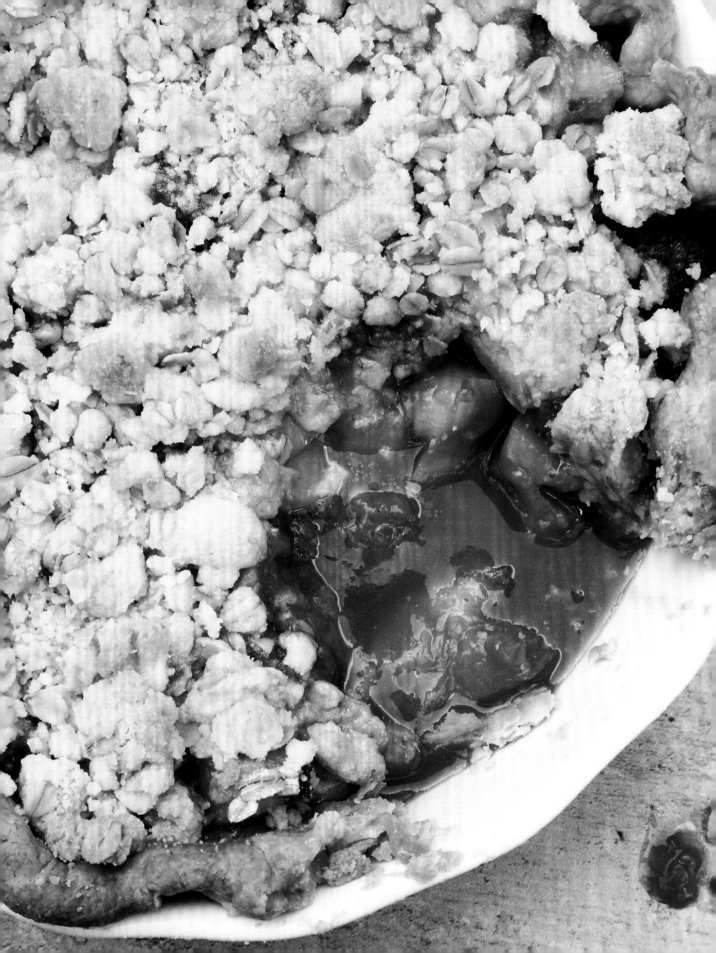

Raspberry and Peach Pie, *continued*

Filling

2 large fresh peaches or 3 cups frozen peaches, cut into ½-inch pieces

¾ cup raspberries

2 tablespoons dark brown sugar

3½ teaspoons granulated sugar

2½ teaspoons cornstarch

2 teaspoons all-purpose flour

2 teaspoons freshly squeezed lemon juice

Line the pie shell with parchment paper and fill with pie weights or dried beans. Bake until the crust is set and the edges are lightly browned, about 45 minutes. Remove from the oven and remove the pie weights and parchment.

In a small bowl, whisk together the egg and egg yolk until blended, then brush the bottom, sides, and edge of the crust with the beaten egg. Return the crust to the oven and bake until golden and firm, about 20 minutes longer. Transfer to a wire rack and let cool completely. You can bake the crust up to a day in advance and then wrap it well and store at room temperature.

To make the oat crumble: In a small saucepan over low heat, warm the butter with the vanilla just until the butter melts, then remove from the heat.

In a medium bowl, stir together the flour, oats, granulated sugar, and salt. Pour the butter mixture into the flour mixture and mix with loose fingertips just until small crumbles form. Transfer to a baking sheet, spread in a thin layer, and chill until firm, about 20 minutes. The crumble can be transferred to a ziplock bag and refrigerated for up to 5 days or frozen for up to 1 month.

Heat the oven to 325°F.

To make the filling: In a large bowl, combine the peaches, raspberries, brown sugar, granulated sugar, cornstarch, flour, and lemon juice and stir to mix evenly.

Spoon the filling into the baked pie crust, then top evenly with the oat crumble.

Bake the pie until the crumble is golden and the filling is bubbling, about 1 hour. Transfer to a wire rack and let cool slightly. The pie will keep, covered, in the refrigerator for up to 5 days. Serve warm or at room temperature.

THC
13.4 mg per serving;
133.8 mg total recipe

Strawberry Shortcake Trifle

MUNCHIES Test Kitchen

Yield: 10 servings

12 egg whites

1 teaspoon kosher salt

1 cup granulated sugar

3 teaspoons vanilla extract

1 cup cake flour

1 cup confectioners' sugar

6 cups thinly sliced strawberries

1½ cups heavy cream

½ cup weed-infused cream
(see page 72)

Angel food cake is super-hard to get weed into because it is so delicate and low in fat. So instead, we've worked the weed into a strawberry shortcake–inspired trifle. This layered confection has delicate cake, sweet juicy strawberries, and weed-loaded whipped cream. Source a strain of weed full of ripe berry notes, like Strawberry Haze or Strawberry Cough, to make your infused cream (and to roll into a joint to pair with your dessert). If you don't feel like spooning from a trifle bowl, layer in individual glasses.

Heat the oven to 325°F.

In a large bowl, using a handheld mixer on medium speed, beat the egg whites and salt until foamy, then increase the speed to medium-high and beat until soft peaks form. Gradually add ⅔ cup of the granulated sugar and continue beating until stiff peaks form. Stir in 2 teaspoons of the vanilla until evenly mixed.

In a medium bowl, stir together the flour and ⅔ cup of the confectioners' sugar. With the mixer on low speed, gradually add one-third of the flour mixture to the egg whites and mix just until incorporated. Repeat with the remaining flour mixture in two equal batches, again mixing just until incorporated after each addition. Pour the batter into a 10-inch tube pan, then bang the pan lightly on the counter to remove any air pockets.

Bake the cake until golden on top and a cake tester or toothpick inserted into the center comes out clean, 25 to 30 minutes.

Remove the cake from the oven and invert the pan to cool. (Most tube pans have small feet attached to the rim, so the pan will stand clear of the work surface when inverted. If your pan doesn't, you will need to improvise. For example, slipping the tube over the neck of a wine bottle works.) Let the cake stand until cooled completely, about 1 hour. Slide a knife around the sides and center tube of the pan to loosen the cake sides, then gently remove the cake from the pan.

continued

Vanessa Says: For added flavor and a boozy kick, macerate the strawberries in weed tequila (see Nitrous Green Dragon, page 77) before adding them to the trifle, or drizzle the fruit with a little of the glycerin-based cannabis tincture on page 83 for some extra THC.

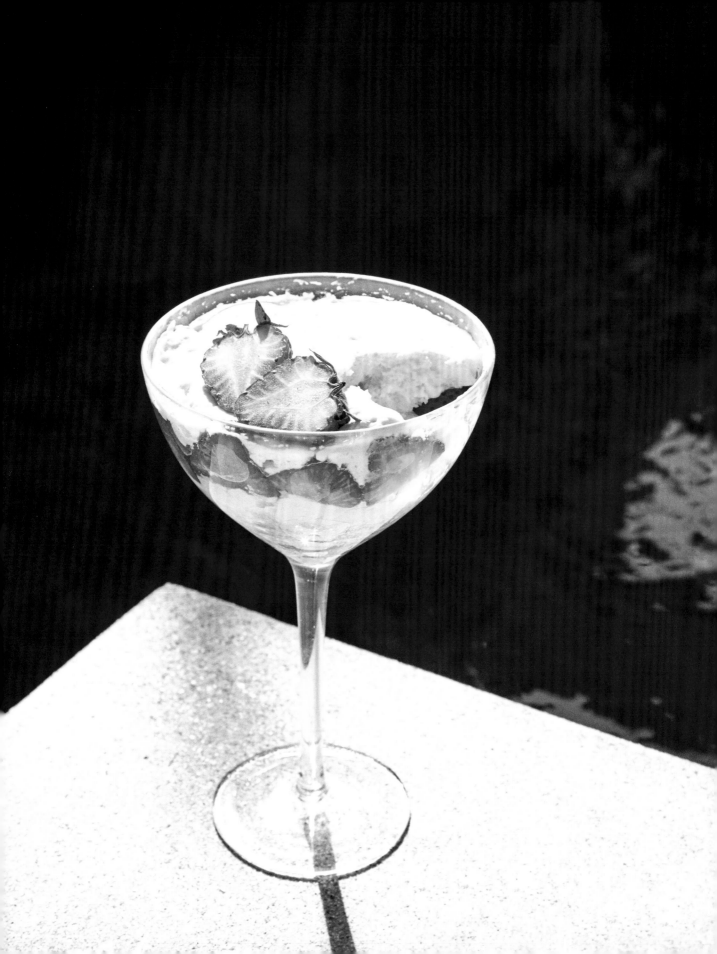

Strawberry Shortcake Trifle, *continued*

In a medium bowl, toss the strawberries with the remaining ⅓ cup granulated sugar. Let sit for 15 minutes, stirring occasionally.

In a large bowl, combine both creams, the remaining ⅓ cup confectioners' sugar, and remaining 1 teaspoon vanilla. Using the handheld mixer or a whisk, beat until the cream is thick and silky. Cover and refrigerate until ready to use, up to 1 day.

Tear the cake into 1-inch pieces. Layer one-third of the cakes pieces on the bottom of a trifle bowl (a 4-quart trifle bowl is traditional, but you can use whatever you have) and top with one-third of the whipped cream. Drizzle with some of the strawberry juice, then spoon about one-third of the strawberries on top. Repeat the layering until you have three layers each of angel food, whipped cream, and strawberries. Cover and refrigerate up to overight, then use a large spoon to serve.

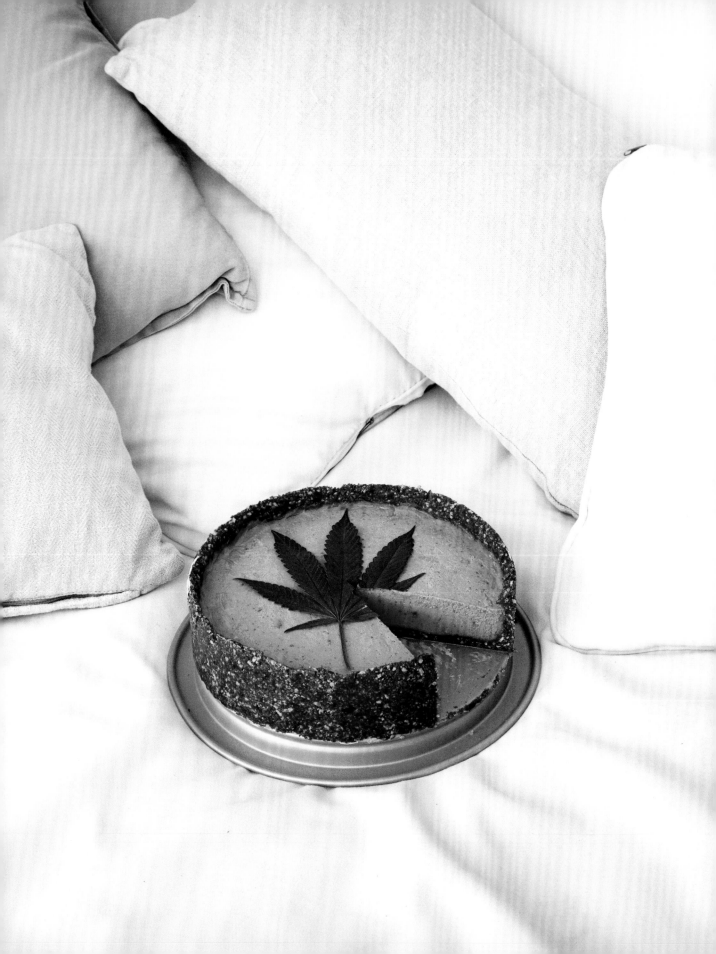

THC

8.9 mg per slice;
71.2 mg total recipe

With weed-infused coconut oil
in the crust: 13.4 mg per slice;
106.8 mg total recipe

Crust

2 cups skin-on raw almonds

10 Medjool dates, pitted

2 tablespoons coconut oil, or flower-infused coconut oil (see page 71)

2 tablespoons raw cacao powder

1 tablespoon kosher salt

Filling

2 cups strawberries, hulled

3 cups raw cashews, soaked in water to cover overnight, then drained and rinsed

1 cup dried goji berries or dried cherries

¾ cup maple syrup

¼ cup freshly squeezed lemon juice

¼ cup coconut butter

¼ cup flower-infused coconut oil (see page 71)

Strawberry "Cheesecake"

Jasmine Shimoda

Yield: 8 equal slices

This is another banger from yogi chef Jasmine Shimoda (see her inspired kale salad on page 124). It's a gluten-free, dairy-free, raw "cheesecake" that is (a) full of weed and (b) genuinely enjoyable. If you can't find sweet-tart goji berries, dried cherries work fine, but the internet works better. A whole fan leaf placed on the top when serving will make the presentation iconic.

To make the crust: Put the almonds in a food processor and pulse until reduced to a fine powder. Add the dates, coconut oil, cacao powder, and salt and process until the dough comes together to form a ball. Transfer the dough to a 9-inch springform pan and press evenly onto the bottom. Cover with plastic wrap and refrigerate for 1 hour.

To make the filling: Place the strawberries in a blender and process until smooth. Add the cashews, goji berries, maple syrup, and lemon juice and process again until smooth. Finally, add the coconut butter and infused coconut oil and process until smooth.

Pour the filling into the springform pan, spreading it evenly over the crust, then cover tightly and freeze for 24 hours. (The cake will keep in the freezer for up to 1 month before serving.)

Release and lift off the pan sides and slide the cake onto a serving plate. Leave to soften slightly in the refrigerator for 1 hour before serving. Any leftovers will keep in the refrigerator for up to 5 days.

Pro Tip: See if you can find a Goji Berry OG Kush strain by Bodhi to make this super soigné.

Bananas Foster

MUNCHIES Test Kitchen

Yield: 4 servings

THC

17.5 mg per serving,
72 mg total recipe

With cannabis flower:
19.9 mg per serving,
81.5 mg total recipe

1½ cups firmly packed light brown sugar

3 tablespoons flower-infused butter (see page 68)

0.5 gram raw kief

½ teaspoon kosher salt

4 bananas, peeled, halved lengthwise, and then halved crosswise into 16 pieces

3 grams cannabis flower (optional)

¼ cup Cognac (preferably Hennessy)

Vanilla ice cream for serving

Classic Bananas Foster is already a fairly dramatic dish, what with the lighting things on fire and all. This version adds a little extra drama with infused butter and kief. And if you're fully prepared to live large, warm some fat nugs in the butter with the bananas and get it all real smoky.

In a 12-inch skillet over medium-low heat, combine the brown sugar, infused butter, kief, and salt and cook, stirring, until the sugar dissolves in the butter. Add the bananas and cannabis flower (if using) and cook, stirring gently every now and again, until the bananas are soft, about 10 minutes.

Add the Cognac, let it heat briefly, and then, working carefully, ignite the Cognac with a long match or a fire starter. Continue to cook until the flames die out. Serve immediately with ice cream.

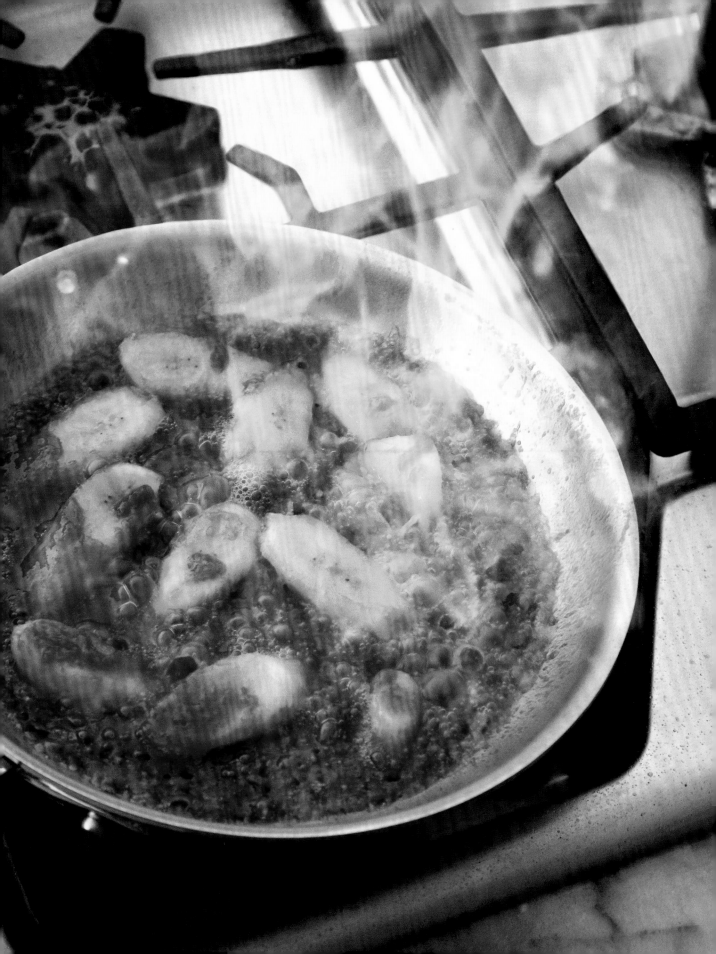

THC
5 mg per gummy;
450 mg total recipe

After-Dinner Mint Gummies

Anna Posey/Elske

Yield: 90 gummies

Vegetable oil for greasing

½ cup confectioners' sugar

½ cup cornstarch

2 cups plus 4 tablespoons water

24 sheets silver gelatin

1½ teaspoons eucalyptus extract

½ teaspoon spearmint extract

½ teaspoon matcha powder

¼ teaspoon spirulina powder

2⅔ cups liquid sucrose

1 tablespoon liquid glucose

½ cup plus 3½ tablespoons glycerin cannabis tincture (see page 83)

2 egg whites

Think of this as a super-classy after-dinner mint that refreshes your palate *and* gets you high (and it gets its color from spirulina, so it can probably cure your cold, too). Pastry chef Anna Posey, of Elske in Chicago, is known for her restrained, delicate nature-inspired desserts, and this deep, deep green eucalyptus-and-mint jelly is no exception. You'll need to hunt down some of the ingredients—stopping at specialty baking and candy supply shops and natural food stores, or the internet for the whole lot—but these sweets are worth the trouble.

Line a 9 by 13-inch sheet pan with parchment paper, then grease the parchment with vegetable oil.

In a small bowl, stir together the confectioners' sugar and cornstarch, mixing well. Dust the prepared pan evenly with ¼ cup of the mixture, then set aside.

Pour 1 cup plus 2 tablespoons of the water into a small saucepan, immerse the gelatin in the water, and let sit until soft, about 5 minutes. Place the pan over medium-low heat and warm just until the gelatin melts, then stir in the eucalyptus extract, spearmint extract, matcha, and spirulina. Remove from the heat and set aside.

In a second small saucepan, stir together the sucrose, glucose, tincture, and remaining 1 cup plus 2 tablespoons water. Place over medium heat and warm without stirring to 260°F on a deep-frying (candy) thermometer. (It is important not to stir while heating as it can cause crystallization.) Remove from the heat, whisk the gelatin mixture into the syrup mixture, and set aside.

Meanwhile, in a medium bowl, whisk the egg whites until frothy. While continuously whisking (by hand or with a handheld mixer), gradually pour the gelatin-syrup mixture in a slow, steady stream into the egg whites. Take care to pour the hot syrup directly into the egg whites, being careful it does not hit the whisk first and splash against the sides of the bowl. (If the syrup spatters, it will adhere to the bowl sides.) Continue to whisk until the mixture has thickened slightly.

Pour the mixture into the prepared pan in an even layer. Dust with ¼ cup confectioners' sugar mixture and let sit at room temperature until set, for about 3 hours.

Dust a cutting board with about 2 tablespoons confectioners' sugar mixture. Cut the gummy sheet into ninety 1 by 1⅓-inch pieces, then remove the pieces from the pan and roll them in the remaining confectioners' sugar mixture, dusting off any excess. Transfer to an airtight container and store at room temperature for up to 2 weeks.

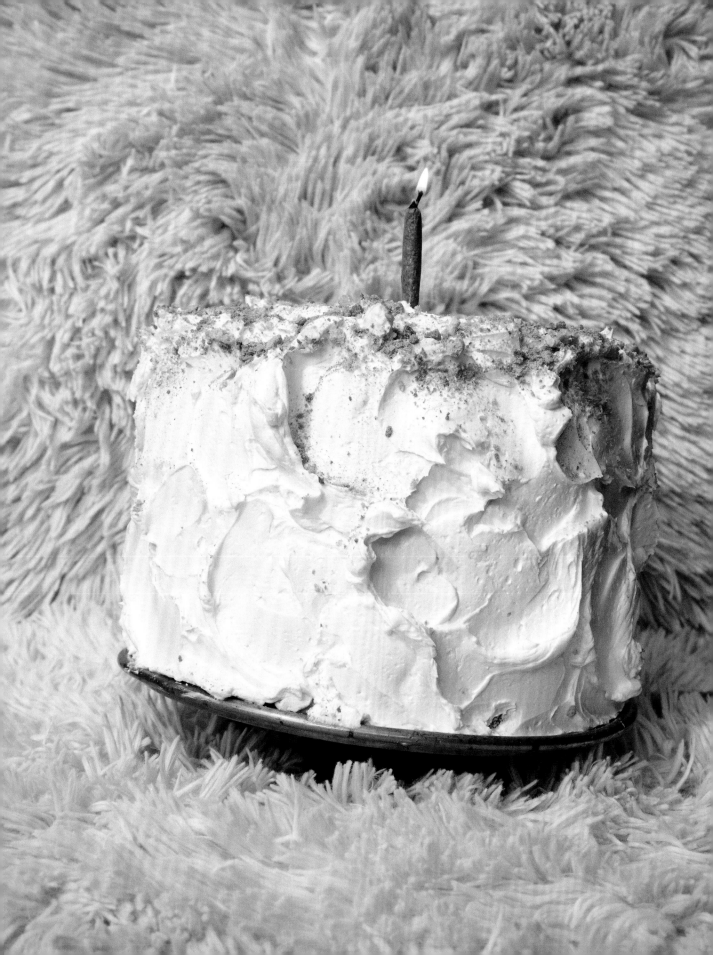

Adult Celebration Cake

Michelle Gayer/Salty Tart

Yield: 16 equal slices

This towering, cream-stuffed, Froot Loops–packed cake from Michelle Gayer of Minneapolis bakery Salty Tart is kind of a brainteaser for the stoner cook: We see at least five places (twice in the cake batter, once in the buttercream, twice in the filling) where you can sneak in some weed. Can you find any others?

	THC IN MILLIGRAMS	
	Per Slice	Total Recipe
with weed-infused olive oil	14.5	233
with weed-infused butter	20.8	334
with weed-infused olive oil and weed-infused butter	35	560

Cake

1 cup olive oil, regular or flower-infused (see page 64)

1 cup sour cream

1¼ cups butter, unsalted or flower-infused (see page 68), at room temperature

5⅔ cups cake flour

3½ cups granulated sugar

¼ cup baking powder

1½ teaspoons kosher salt

3 cups whole milk

7 large eggs, lightly beaten

1 cup Fruit Loops cereal, chopped

Heat the oven to 350°F. Grease three 8-inch round cake pans, then line the bottoms with parchment paper.

In a stand mixer fitted with the paddle attachment, combine the olive oil, sour cream, and butter. Top with the flour, sugar, baking powder, and salt. Mix on medium speed just until a crumbly consistency forms. In a medium bowl, whisk together the milk and eggs until blended. With the mixer on low speed, slowly add the milk-egg mixture in three equal additions, mixing until fully combined and scraping down the sides of the bowl after each addition. With the mixer still on low speed, add the cereal and mix just until combined. Divide the batter evenly among the prepared cake pans.

Bake the cakes until a knife inserted into the center of one comes out clean, about 55 minutes. Transfer to wire racks and let cool for about 20 minutes. Run a knife blade around the inside edge of a pan to loosen the cake sides, invert the cake onto a rack, lift off the pan, peel off the parchment, and turn the layer right-side up. Repeat with

continued

Adult Celebration Cake, *continued*

the remaining cakes and let cool completely. The cakes can be well wrapped and stored at room temperature for up to 3 days or in the freezer for up to 1 month; thaw overnight in the refrigerator.

Buttercream

3¼ cups granulated sugar

14 egg whites

4 cups unsalted butter, plus 6 tablespoons, unsalted or flower-infused (see page 68), at room temperature

6 tablespoons hot water

1 teaspoon kosher salt

Grated zest of 1 lemon

	THC IN MILLIGRAMS	
	Per Slice	Total Recipe
with weed-infused butter	6.3	100

Pour water to a depth of 1 inch in a 4-quart saucepan and bring to a simmer over medium heat. Put the sugar and egg whites in a large heatproof bowl and set the bowl over (not touching) the water in the saucepan. Heat, stirring, until the sugar has dissolved into the egg whites, about 10 minutes.

Transfer the egg white–sugar mixture to the stand mixer fitted with the whisk attachment and whisk on medium-high speed until cool and thick. Add the butter and continue to whisk until creamy and thick. Add the hot water, salt, and lemon zest and whisk until fully incorporated, about 3 minutes longer. Cover and refrigerate for up to 1 week.

Whipped Cream Filling

1 cup heavy cream, plus 1 cup, heavy or weed-infused (see page 72)

1 cup sour cream

¾ cup whipped honey, regular or weed-infused (see page 74)

1 pinch kosher salt

	THC IN MILLIGRAMS	
	Per Slice	Total Recipe
with weed-infused cream	33.4	535
with whipped weed-infused honey	1.6	56
with weed-infused cream and whipped weed-infused honey	35	560`

In the stand mixer fitted with the whisk attachment, combine the heavy cream, sour cream, honey, and salt and whisk on high speed until thick and fluffy, 5 to 8 minutes. Cover and refrigerate for up to 3 days.

Froot Loops for sprinkling

Using a long, serrated knife in a sawing motion, horizontally split each cake into three layers. To make it easier to cut, freeze the cakes for about 2 hours before cutting into thirds. You will have a total of nine layers.

Set a cake layer on a cake plate. Spoon about one-fourth of the buttercream into a piping bag fitted with a ½-inch plain tip and pipe a narrow wall around the edge of the layer (this is a "fence" to keep the cream filling in place). Fill the center with about ½ cup of the filling, spreading it in an even layer with an offset spatula. Top with a second cake layer and repeat the fence and filling. Continue in this way until you have stacked and filled eight layers. Top with the final cake layer and, using the offset spatula, spread a thin layer of buttercream over the top and sides of the cake to seal in any loose crumbs, creating a smooth surface. Refrigerate the cake for about 30 minutes to set the crumb coat.

To finish, mound about one-third of the remaining buttercream on top of the cake and, using broad, smooth strokes, spread it evenly. Then, working in batches, apply the remaining buttercream to the sides of the cake in an even layer, returning to the top once again to smooth any rough edges. Sprinkle the top with Froot Loops. The cake will keep, covered, in the refrigerator, for up to 5 days. Cut into even slices to serve.

Choose-Your-Own-Adventure Assembly

	THC IN MILLIGRAMS	
	Per Slice	Total Recipe
Buttercream with weed-infused butter and Filling with weed-infused cream	39.6	635
Buttercream with weed-infused butter and Filling with whipped weed-infused honey	7.8	125.6
Buttercream with weed-infused butter and Filling with weed-infused cream and whipped weed-infused honey	41.3	660

	THC IN MILLIGRAMS	
	Per Slice	Total Recipe
Cake with weed-infused olive oil and Buttercream with weed-infused butter	20.8	333
Cake with weed-infused butter and Buttercream with weed-infused butter	27	434
Cake with weed-infused olive oil and weed-infused butter and Buttercream with weed-infused butter	41.6	665

Vanessa Says: A cake of this measure deserves the appropriate accessories. Candied cannabis leaves are crunchy and sweet. Lay smaller fan leaves on a parchment-lined baking sheet and paint them with a 3:1 sugar-to-water simple syrup. Place in a 240°F oven for 10 minutes (ideally with convection; it'll take a little longer without), until glossy and dry.

continued

Adult Celebration Cake, *continued*

	THC IN MILLIGRAMS	
	Per Slice	Total Recipe
Cake with weed-infused olive oil and Filling with weed-infused cream	47.9	766
Cake with weed-infused olive oil and Filling with whipped weed-infused honey	16	257
Cake with weed-infused olive oil and Filling with weed-infused cream and whipped weed-infused honey	50	790

	THC IN MILLIGRAMS	
	Per Slice	Total Recipe
Cake with weed-infused butter and Filling with weed-infused cream	54	867
Cake with weed-infused butter and Filling with whipped weed-infused honey	22.4	358
Cake with weed-infused butter and Filling with weed-infused cream and whipped weed-infused honey	55.6	889.6

	THC IN MILLIGRAMS	
	Per Slice	Total Recipe
Cake with weed-infused olive oil and weed-infused butter and Filling with weed-infused cream	68.7	1,099
Cake with weed-infused olive oil and weed-infused butter and Filling with whipped weed-infused honey	37	590
Cake with weed-infused olive oil and weed-infused butter and Filling with weed-infused cream and whipped weed-infused honey	70	1,125

	THC IN MILLIGRAMS	
	Per Slice	Total Recipe
Cake with weed-infused olive oil, Buttercream with weed-infused butter, and Filling with weed-infused cream	54	864
Cake with weed-infused olive oil, Buttercream with weed-infused butter, and Filling with whipped weed-infused honey	22.4	357
Cake with weed-infused olive oil, Buttercream with weed-infused butter, and Filling with weed-infused cream and whipped weed-infused honey	55.7	892

	THC IN MILLIGRAMS	
	Per Slice	Total Recipe
Cake with weed-infused butter, Buttercream with weed-infused butter, and Filling with weed-infused cream	60	967
Cake with weed-infused butter, Buttercream with weed-infused butter, and Filling with whipped weed-infused honey	28.6	458
Cake with weed-infused butter, Buttercream with weed-infused butter, and Filling with weed-infused cream and whipped weed-infused honey	61.6	985

	THC IN MILLIGRAMS	
	Per Slice	Total Recipe
Cake with weed-infused olive oil and weed-infused butter, Buttercream with weed-infused butter, and Filling with weed-infused cream	75	1,200
Cake with weed-infused olive oil and weed-infused butter, Buttercream with weed-infused butter, and Filling with whipped weed-infused honey	43	688
Cake with weed-infused olive oil and weed-infused butter, Buttercream with weed-infused butter, and Filling with weed-infused cream and whipped weed-infused honey	76.5	1,225

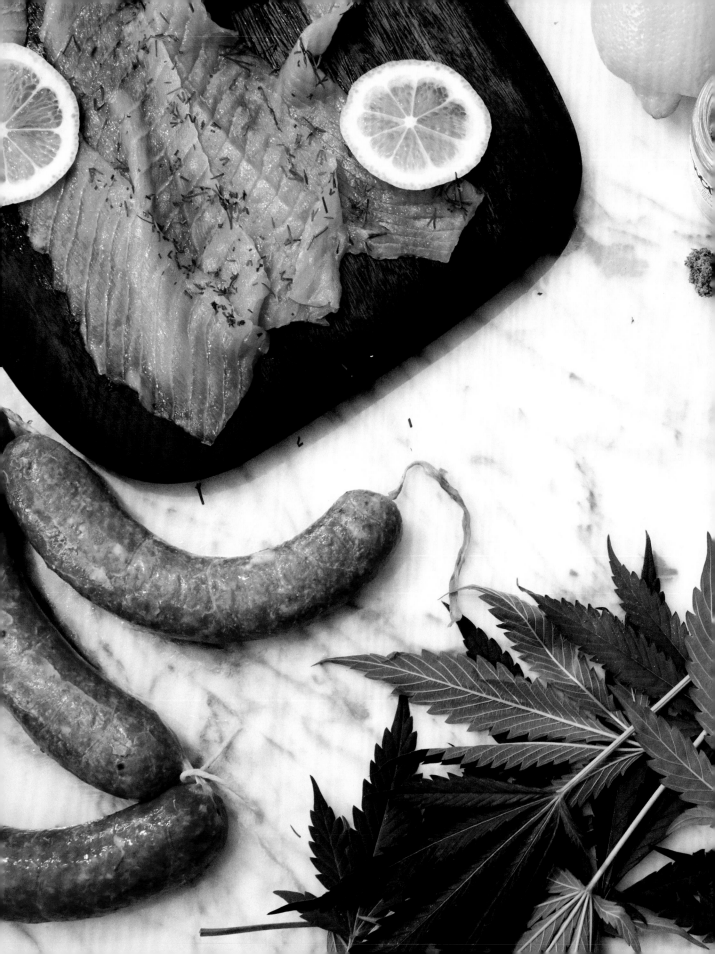

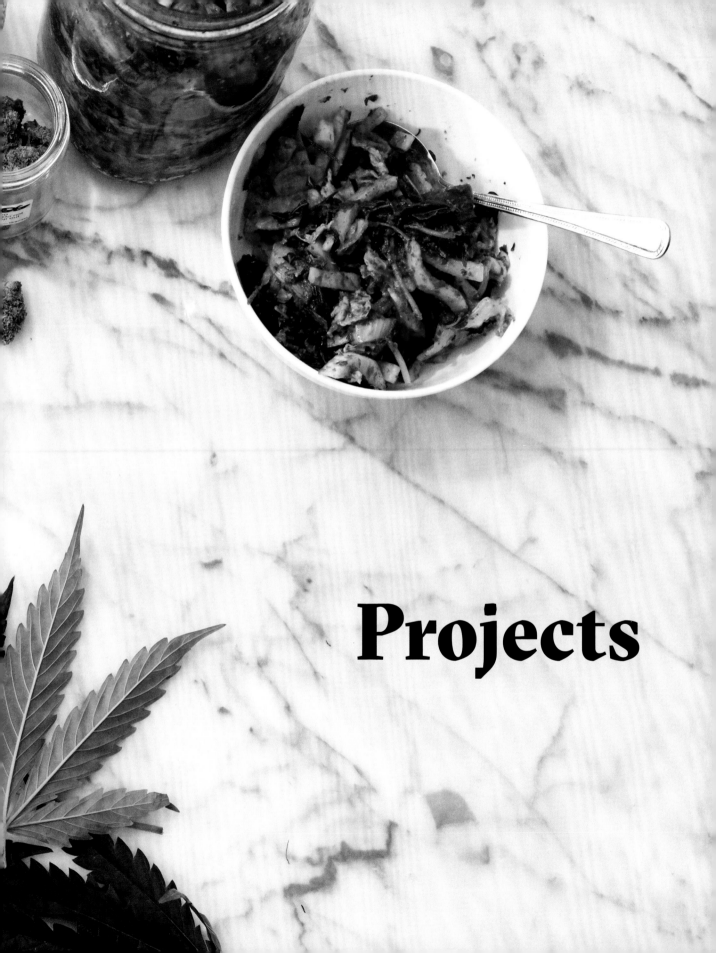

Projects

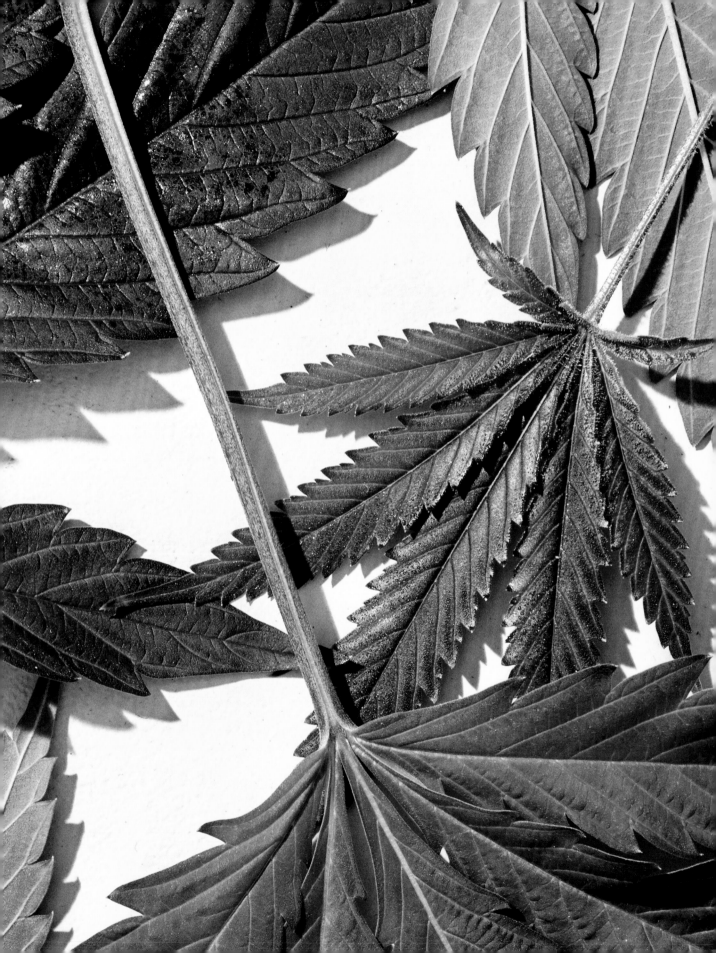

THC
20.8 mg per ¼ cup;
83.2 mg total recipe

Cannabis Leaf Pesto

MUNCHIES Test Kitchen

Yield: 1 cup

4 cannabis fan leaves

1½ cups basil leaves

¼ cup pine nuts, toasted

½ cup grated Parmesan cheese

**½ cup flower-infused olive oil
(see page 64)**

Kosher salt

Much as in the chimichurri on page 157, weed leaves add vegetal vibes to this classic pesto. If you want to make things extra soigné, chilling the olive oil for a half hour in the fridge before adding it to the pesto helps the leaves stay nice and green while they're being pulverized.

In a food processor, combine the cannabis leaves, basil, pine nuts, cheese, and infused olive oil and process all of the leaves all finely chopped. Season with salt. Use right away, or transfer to an airtight container and store in the refrigerator for up to 3 days.

THC
1.3 mg per serving;
5.3 mg total recipe

Cannabis Leaf Chips

MUNCHIES Test Kitchen

Yield: 4 servings

1¼ pounds cannabis fan leaves

1½ teaspoons flower-infused olive oil (see page 64)

Kosher salt

Save the kale chips for precious Brooklyn toddlers and chow down on pot-leaf chips instead. No, they won't get you high on their own (that's what the infused olive oil is for), but it still wouldn't kill you to eat some greens. In fact, it would do you some good. Cannabis, just like all those other leafy greens, is loaded with protein, fiber, vitamins C and K, folate, iron, antioxidants, and more.

Heat the oven to 300°F. Line two large baking sheets with parchment paper.

Divide the cannabis leaves among the prepared baking sheets, drizzle evenly with the infused olive oil, and then massage the oil gently into the leaves. Spread the leaves into a single layer and season generously with salt.

Bake the leaves until crispy, 10 to 12 minutes. Let cool to room temperature before serving. Store in an airtight container at room temperature for up to 3 days.

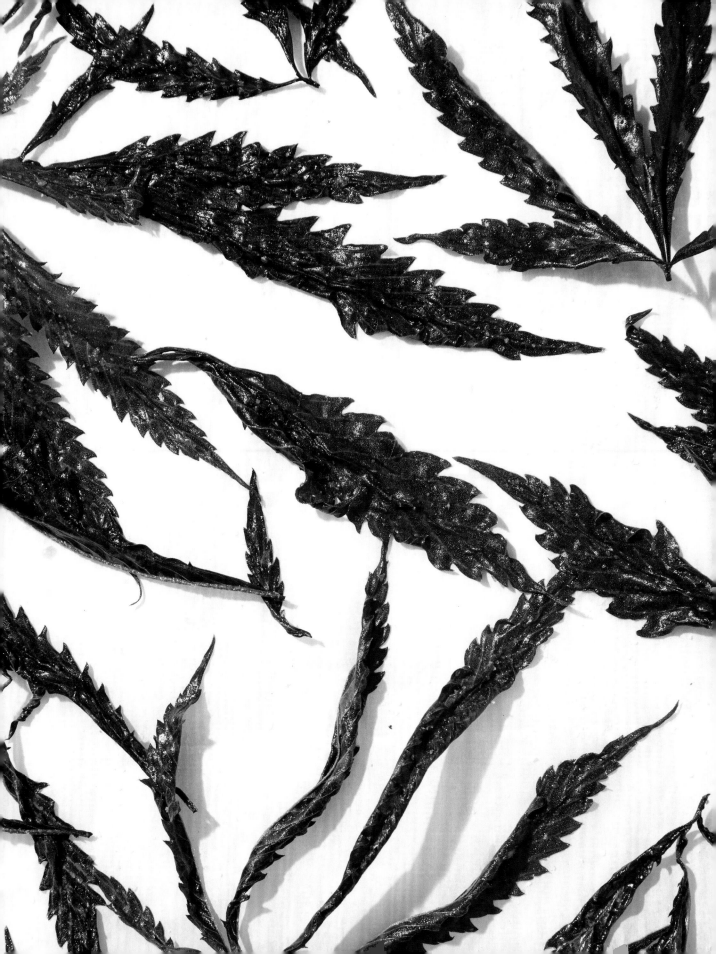

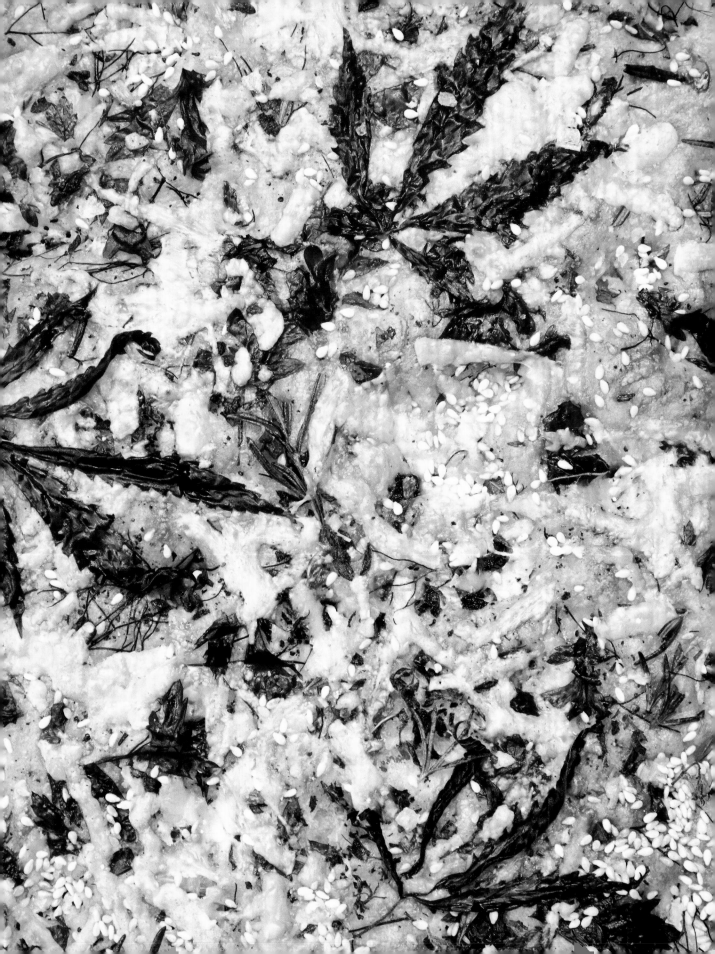

THC
5.2 mg per serving;
62.4 mg total

Herb Focaccia

MUNCHIES Test Kitchen

Yield: 12 servings

¾ cup hot (115°F) water

One ¼-ounce packet active dry yeast

½ teaspoon granulated sugar

1¾ cups all-purpose flour

Kosher salt

6 tablespoons flower-infused olive oil (see page 64)

½ cup dill leaves

½ cup fresh mint leaves

½ cup fresh parsley leaves

¼ cup fresh oregano leaves

¼ cup fresh rosemary leaves

2 garlic cloves, minced

Freshly ground black pepper

Freshly squeezed lemon juice for seasoning

Cannabis leaves for decorating (optional)

½ cup grated Parmesan cheese

2 tablespoons sesame seeds

Focaccia is deceptively easy; all you have to do is stir the ingredients together, ignore them for a while, then bake, and you end up with a perfectly bubbly, soft-on-the-inside and lightly-fried-on-the-outside flatbread. This particular version is topped with Parmesan, a ton of fresh herbs and fresh *herb*. It will keep in an airtight container for up to 5 days at room temperature and is especially good with the Homemade Ricotta Cheese on page 233, or dunked in olive oil, either infused or regular.

In the bowl of a stand mixer fitted with the dough hook, combine the water, yeast, and sugar and let sit until foamy, about 10 minutes. Add the flour and ½ teaspoon salt and then mix on medium speed until a smooth dough forms, about 5 minutes. Cover the bowl with plastic wrap and let the dough rise for 30 minutes.

Drizzle 2 tablespoons of the infused olive oil on a 9 by 13-inch sheet pan.

Once the dough has risen, using your fingers and hands, stretch it into the prepared pan. Stretch and dimple the dough over the course of the next hour to ensure it's the size of the pan (keep it covered with plastic wrap when you're not dimpling it).

In a food processor, combine the dill, mint, parsley, oregano, rosemary, and garlic and pulse to mix. Season with 1½ teaspoons salt, 1½ teaspoons pepper, and lemon juice, then stream in the remaining 4 tablespoons infused oil until you have a perfect loose paste with which to top your dough.

Top the dough with the herb paste, decorate with cannabis leaves, and sprinkle with the Parmesan, sesame seeds, and salt and pepper. Let rise for about 45 minutes.

Heat the oven to 425°F.

Using your fingers, gently press dimples into the surface of the dough, then bake until golden brown, about 20 minutes. Let cool slightly, then cut into 12 slices and serve.

THC
8.3 mg per roll;
133.6 mg total recipe

Dinner Rolls

Timothy Hollingsworth/Otium
Yield: 16 rolls

Rolls

½ cup lukewarm (110°F) water

2¼ teaspoons active dry yeast

4 cups all-purpose flour

¼ cup granulated sugar

1½ teaspoons kosher salt

½ cup whole milk

4 tablespoons flower-infused butter (see page 68), melted

1 large egg, lightly beaten

2 tablespoons olive oil

Egg Wash

2 egg yolks

3 tablespoons water

1 teaspoon kosher salt

From chef Timothy Hollingsworth of L.A.'s Otium restaurant come these soft, pillowy dinner rolls ideal for stuffing carbs into your face. Brushing infused butter on these rolls is a hella easy way to add weed to any meal without going to a whole lot of trouble. Leftover rolls will keep in an airtight container, at room temperature, for up to 3 days.

To make the rolls: Put the warm water in the bowl of a stand mixer fitted with the dough hook attachment and stir in the yeast. Let stand until foamy, about 10 minutes. Meanwhile, in a medium bowl, stir together the flour, sugar, and salt.

Add the flour mixture, milk, infused butter, and egg to the mixer bowl and beat on low speed for 5 minutes. Increase the speed to medium-high and beat until the dough is smooth and elastic, about 5 minutes longer.

Grease a large bowl with 1 tablespoon of the olive oil. Gather up the dough, shape into a ball, transfer to the oiled bowl, and turn the dough to coat all sides with oil. Cover the bowl with plastic wrap and let the dough rise in a warm area until it doubles in size, about 1 hour. Punch the dough down, re-cover the bowl, and refrigerate for 1 hour longer.

Grease a 12-inch cast-iron skillet with the remaining 1 tablespoon olive oil. Portion the dough into sixteen equal balls and nestle them, not touching, in the skillet. Cover loosely with plastic wrap and let rise in a warm area until the rolls have doubled in size, about 1 hour.

To make the egg wash: In a small bowl, whisk together the egg yolks, water, and salt. Set aside.

Herb Butter

4 tablespoons flower-infused butter (see page 68), melted

1 tablespoon minced fresh thyme

1 tablespoon crushed Aleppo pepper

1 garlic clove, minced

Grated zest of 1 lemon

Freshly ground black pepper

Maldon sea salt

Vanessa Says: Use a herbaceous, piney strain of weed, like Jack Herer or Romulan, to infuse the butter for these rolls. Up the THC dose (and add a nice shine) by brushing more infused butter on top.

To make the herb butter: In a small bowl, whisk together the infused butter, thyme, Aleppo pepper, garlic, and lemon zest and season with black pepper. Set aside.

Heat the oven to 350°F.

Brush the tops of the rolls with the egg wash, then sprinkle each roll with a small pinch of Maldon salt.

Bake the rolls for 20 minutes. Remove the skillet from the oven and brush the tops of the rolls with all of the herb butter, dividing it evenly. Return the skillet to the oven and bake until the rolls are golden brown on top, about 10 minutes longer. Serve warm.

THC
8.4 mg per serving;
100 mg total recipe

Corn Biscuits

Zoe Taylor/Milktooth

Yield: 12 biscuits

3⅔ cups all-purpose flour

1 tablespoon kosher salt

1 teaspoon baking soda

6 tablespoons flower-infused butter (see page 68), frozen and grated on the large holes of a box grater

6 tablespoons unsalted butter, frozen and grated on the large holes of a box grater

¾ cup buttermilk

¾ cup sour cream

1 cup fresh or frozen corn kernels

At Milktooth in Indianapolis, Zoe Taylor folds grilled corn kernels into her otherwise super-classic buttermilk biscuits, which gives them a little sweetness, a little smoke, and a little texture. Here, we're amplifying the sweetness with fresh corn (though frozen works too). Zoe's lightly infused cherry elderberry jam (see page 230) makes the biscuits late-summer appropriate; if it's any other season, the weed-infused honey on page 74 ups the ante nicely. Leftover biscuits will keep in an airtight container, at room temperature, for up to 5 days.

Heat the oven to 375°F. Line a baking sheet with parchment paper and set aside.

In a large bowl, stir together the flour, salt, and baking soda. Scatter both butters over the top and, using your fingers, mix the butters with the flour mixture just until pea-size crumbles form. Add the buttermilk and sour cream and mix with your hands just until combined, taking care not to overmix. Stir in the corn kernels.

Turn the dough out onto a lightly floured work surface. Pat into a large rectangle ¾ inch thick and then fold over onto itself five or six times (this helps create the flaky layers that we know and love about biscuits). Pat the dough out again about ¾ inch thick. Using a 2½-inch round biscuit cutter, cut out twelve biscuits, pressing straight down and pulling straight up to form them. Do not twist the cutter as you lift or you will mess up all those buttery, flaky layers you created by folding the dough over onto itself. As the biscuits are cut, transfer them to the prepared baking sheet, spacing them about 1 inch apart.

Bake the biscuits until golden brown, about 15 minutes and rotating the pan 180 degrees halfway through baking. Serve warm.

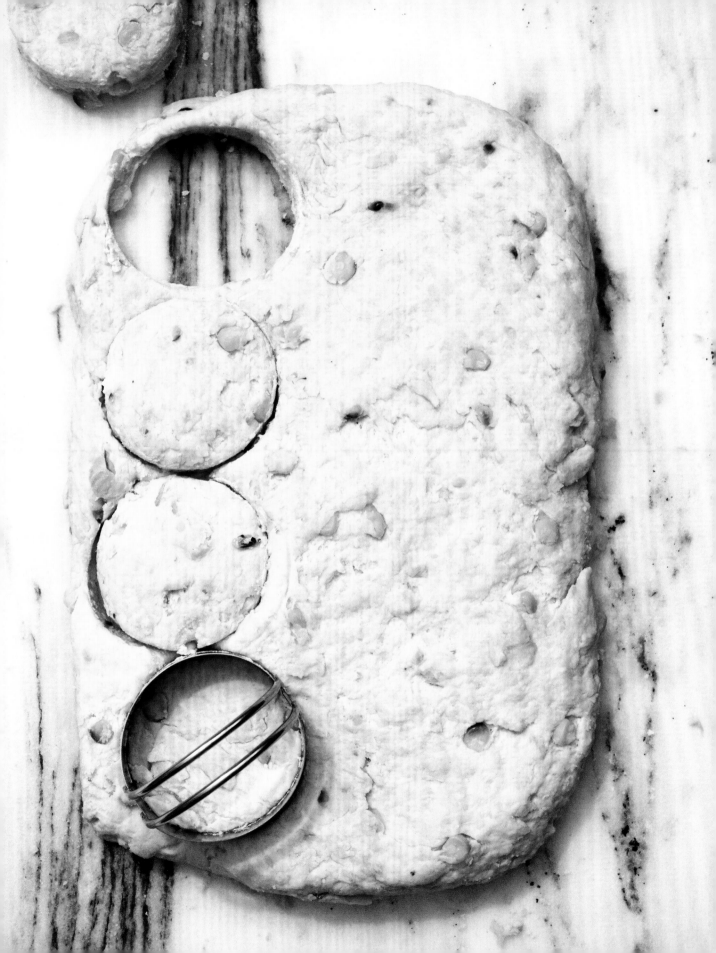

THC

2.6 mg per lemon;
20.8 mg total recipe

Preserved Lemons

Joan Nathan

Yield: 8 lemons

8 lemons, plus 1 cup freshly
squeezed lemon juice, or as
needed

1 cup kosher salt

2 grams cannabis flowers, fresh
or dried and cured

2 tablespoons flower-infused
olive oil (see page 64)

Preserved lemons are a North African pantry staple used to brighten stews, sauces, and salads. This version, which includes a couple of spoonfuls of infused olive oil and some buds, promises to brighten your day, too. Most of the infused oil will remain in the lemony brine, which can be repurposed into an ingredient for salad dressing. If giving as a gift, make the jar decorative by arranging a few fan leaves around the perimeter.

Wash a large canning jar and lid with hot, soapy water, then sterilize them by submerging in boiling water for 30 to 60 seconds. Drain well, transfer to a work surface, and let air-dry.

Cut a thin slice off both ends of each lemon. Quarter each lemon lengthwise, cutting only three-fourths of the way through, so the base remains intact. Pack 2 tablespoons of the salt inside each lemon, pushing the salt into the crevices, and then press the lemon closed. Pack the stuffed lemons into the sterilized jar, layering in the cannabis flowers as you go. The lemons should fit snugly in the jar. Finally, pour in the lemon juice, immersing the lemons in the juice. Screw on the lid and set the jar aside in a cool place for 1 day.

The next day, add the infused olive oil, recap the jar, and then turn it upside down to distribute the oil evenly. Place the jar in the refrigerator and leave to cure for 2 to 3 weeks, until the peels are tender to the bite. The cured lemons will keep, in the refrigerator, for up to 3 months.

Rinse the salt from the lemons before using, then scrape off the pulp (or not if you prefer) and use the peel.

Note: You can shorten the curing period by about 2 weeks by freezing the lemons (pack them into a plastic freezer bag) for a few days after you quarter them. Freezing alters the flesh and peel to speed the penetration of the salt. Thaw and cure with the salt and other ingredients as directed.

Vanessa Says: We threw some fresh buds in here for fun and flavor. Pick a variety high in limonene (such as Super Lemon Haze) or add some herbaceous notes with Jack Herer.

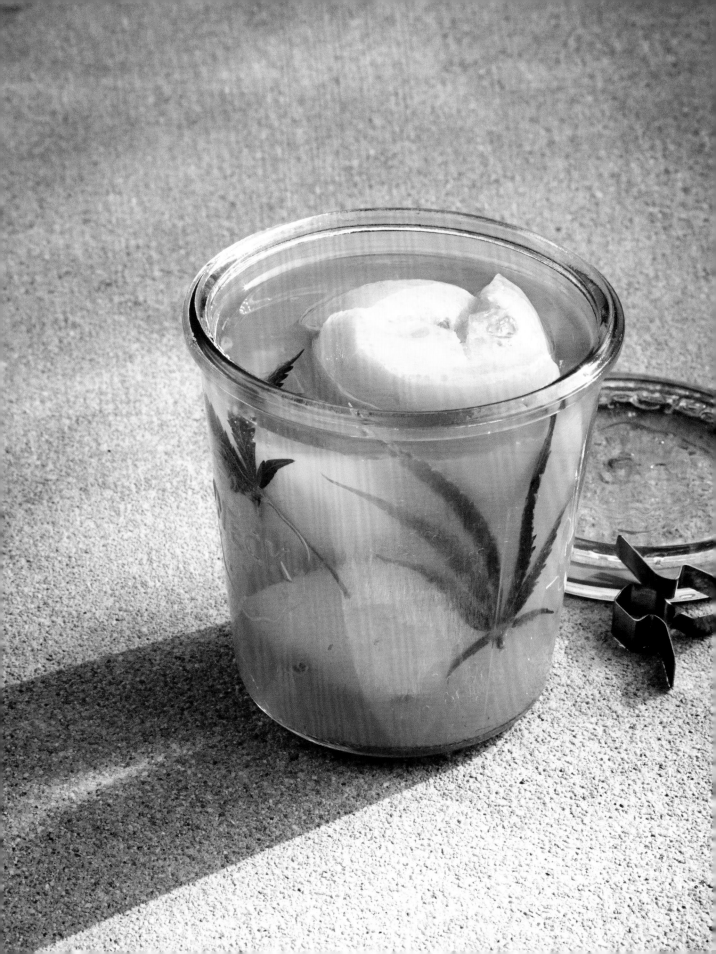

THC

0.8 mg per 2 tablespoons;
39.1 mg total recipe

Cherry Elderberry Jam

Zoe Taylor/Milktooth

Yield: 6½ cups

2 pounds dark, sweet cherries, pitted and halved (pits reserved)

4 cups granulated sugar

2 fresh bay leaves

1 cinnamon stick

1 tablespoon glycerin cannabis tincture (see page 83)

4 cups elderberry juice

¼ cup powdered apple pectin

2 vanilla beans, split lengthwise

Kosher salt

Freshly squeezed lemon juice for seasoning

This is a low-dose spread for slathering on corn biscuits (see page 226) but also for dressing up your morning toast or anything else you might like. You will need three 1-pint canning jars with flat lids and screw bands for storing. (The remaining ½ cup jam can be kept in a covered container in the refrigerator.) Wash the jars and lids in hot, soapy water, then sterilize the jars by immersing in gently boiling water for 10 minutes, and covering the flat lids with boiling water off the heat. Remove the jars from the boiling water, draining them well, just before you are ready to fill them. Have the lids and screw bands ready.

A well-stocked health food store should have both the elderberry juice and the apple pectin (which helps jam solidify).

In a large saucepan over medium-low heat, combine the cherries and 2 cups of the sugar and cook, stirring often to prevent scorching, until the cherries are soft, about 5 minutes. While the cherries cook, put the reserved cherry pits, bay leaves, and cinnamon stick on a piece of cheesecloth and tie together the corners to make a sachet.

When the cherries are soft, add the sachet to the pan along with the remaining 2 cups sugar, the tincture, elderberry juice, and pectin. Using the tip of a knife, scrape the seeds from the vanilla beans, then add the seeds and the pods to the pan. Increase the heat to medium-high and bring to a boil. Turn the heat to a simmer and cook, stirring occasionally, until the mixture is thick and shiny, about 30 minutes. Season with salt and lemon juice.

Place a wire rack in the bottom of a large, tall stockpot, fill the pot three-fourths full of water, and bring to a boil.

Ladle the jam into hot, sterilized jars, leaving ¼-inch headspace, and wipe away any drips from the rim with a damp towel. Top each jar with a flat lid and twist on a screw band. Using jar tongs, lower the jars into the stockpot. The jars should not be touching one another and should be covered by 1 inch of water. Return the water to a

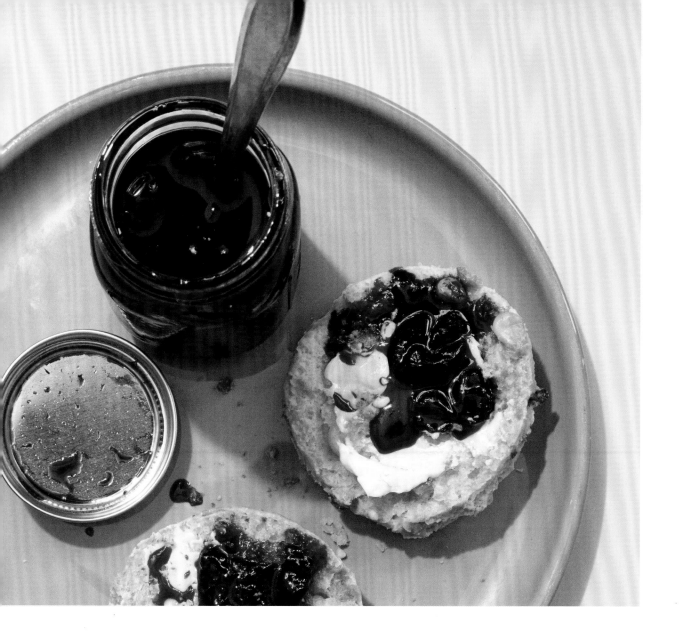

rolling boil, cover, and process for 10 minutes. Turn off the heat, let cool for a few minutes, then, using tongs, transfer the jars to a rack or a towel-lined work surface and let cool completely.

To check if the seal is good on each jar, press against the center of the lid with a fingertip. If the lid remains concave when you remove your finger, the seal is good; if the lid springs back, the seal failed and the jar must be stored in the refrigerator. Jars with a good seal can be stored in a cool, dark place for up to 1 year. Once a jar has been opened, store it in the refrigerator, where it will keep for up to 3 months.

THC
9.2 mg per 2 tablespoons;
110.7 mg total recipe

Homemade Peanut Butter

Melissa D'Elia

Yield: 1½ cups

2 cups unsalted raw peanuts

5 tablespoons flower-infused peanut or vegetable oil (see page 64)

¼ cup whipped weed-infused honey (see page 74)

Kosher salt

This pot-laced peanut butter from cannabis chef Melissa D'Elia is amazingly easy and ridiculously good in both sweet and savory dishes, like the sauce for the Brownie Sundae on page 195 and the Peanut Butter Noodles on page 146, as well as on those nights where all you can manage to make for yourself is a PB&J. Don't be lazy and skip the peanut-roasting step—it gives the finished peanut butter a deeper flavor and smoother texture.

Heat the oven to 350°F.

Spread the peanuts in a single layer on a baking sheet and roast until lightly golden and glossy, 7 to 8 minutes. Remove from the oven and let cool until slightly warm.

Transfer the warm peanuts to a food processor and process for 1 minute. Stop the processor and scrape down the sides and along the bottom of the bowl. The peanut butter will be granular and look a bit like wet sand. Repeat the 1-minute processing and scraping four or five times, until the peanut butter begins to look glossy. Drizzle in the infused peanut oil and honey, sprinkle with salt, and purée until smooth. Taste and adjust the seasoning if needed.

Transfer the peanut butter to an airtight container and store in the refrigerator for up to 6 weeks.

THC
4 mg per 1 tablespoon;
192 mg total recipe

Homemade Ricotta Cheese

Frank Pinello/Best Pizza

Yield: 3 cups

2 quarts whole milk

1 cup weed-infused cream
(see page 72)

½ teaspoon kosher salt

3 tablespoons freshly squeezed
lemon juice

Owner of Best Pizza in Brooklyn, just a stone's throw from the offices of VICE, and host of *The Pizza Show* on MUNCHIES, Frank Pinello is a friend and a damn fine *pizzaiolo* (a person who makes pizzas), as we can testify from having eaten many a slice. His ricotta is—as expected—killer in the Summer Tomato and Stone Fruit Salad on page 120 or the French Bread Pizza on page 110, but maybe even better with a spoon, on your couch, by yourself.

Line a large strainer with cheesecloth and place over a large bowl.

In a medium saucepan over medium heat, combine the milk, infused cream, and salt and bring just to a boil, stirring constantly to prevent scorching. Turn the heat to a low simmer, add the lemon juice, and cook until the mixture curdles and separates into clumps of milky-white curds and thin ivory whey, about 10 minutes. Remove from the heat.

Slowly pour the contents of the pan into the prepared strainer (it can splash if you work too quickly), let drain for 1 hour, and then discard the whey.

Transfer the ricotta to an airtight container and store in the refrigerator for up to 2 days.

THC
10 mg per ½ cup;
80 mg total recipe

Cannabis Kimchi

Holden Jagger/Altered Plates
Yield: 1 quart

1 pound cannabis fan leaves, soaked in water to cover

1 pound napa cabbage, cut into 1-inch pieces

¼ cup Korean sea salt

6 garlic cloves, grated

1 tablespoon peeled and grated ginger

1 gram cannabis flower, ground and decarboxylated (see page 55)

3 tablespoons kelp powder

4 tablespoons Korean red pepper powder (gochugaru)

½ pound Korean radish (mu) or daikon radish, peeled and julienned

4 green onions, white and tender green parts, cut into ¼-inch pieces

Cannabis adds subtle dankness to already-funky kimchi. Fresh leaves won't get you high, but they will add THCA to your diet—call it an herbal supplement. The decarb'ed bud is what delivers the potency here, plus it amps up the weed flavor. Holden Jagger is a private chef who grows his own weed and loves experimenting with plant parts. Know that cannabis leaves are deceptively lightweight, so a pound of them will be more than you might think. After you harvest the leaves, immediately submerge them in water to keep them from wilting. They can be stored this way overnight, either refrigerated or at room temperature. For the Korean-specific ingredients, depending on where you live, visit a Korean market or shop online.

Remove the cannabis leaves from the water and cut them into ½-inch slices. If using large fan leaves, feel free to add some of the stem as well; it will add another level of texture.

In a large bowl, mix together the cannabis leaves and cabbage and pour in the salt. With clean or gloved hands, massage the salt into the vegetables until they soften and begin to release their liquid. Cover the bowl and let the mixture sit at room temperature for 2 hours.

Meanwhile, wash a 1-quart widemouthed canning jar and lid with hot, soapy water, then sterilize by submerging them in boiling water for 30 to 60 seconds. Drain well, transfer to a work surface, and let air-dry.

In a small bowl, combine the garlic, ginger, cannabis flower, kelp powder, and red pepper powder and stir to form a paste.

When the 2 hours are up, transfer the cannabis-cabbage mixture to a colander and rinse under cool running water. Wring out the vegetables, expelling as much liquid as possible. Rinse the large bowl, then return the vegetables to it. Add the radish, green onions, and spice paste, then don gloves and use your hands to mix everything together, working vigorously.

Leaving the gloves on, carefully fill the sterilized jar with the mixture, leaving 1-inch headspace. Loosely screw on the sterilized lid. Do *not* tighten the lid, as an airtight seal can create pressure as the kimchi ferments, causing the jar to explode.

Leave the jar in a cool, dry place out of direct sunlight. The jar will release some interesting aromas as it ferments over the next 5 days, but that's part of the magic! After 5 days, the kimchi should be nice and ripe and the jar will have filled with liquid. Tighten the lid and refrigerate for up to 3 months.

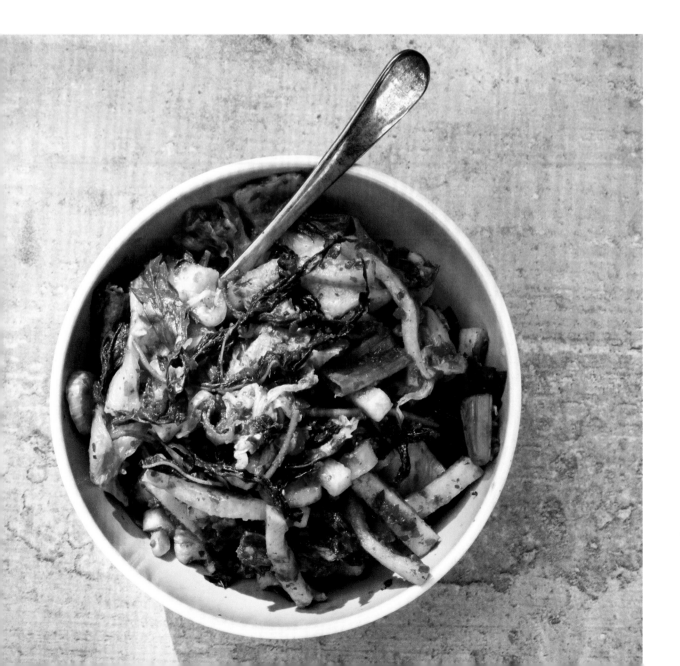

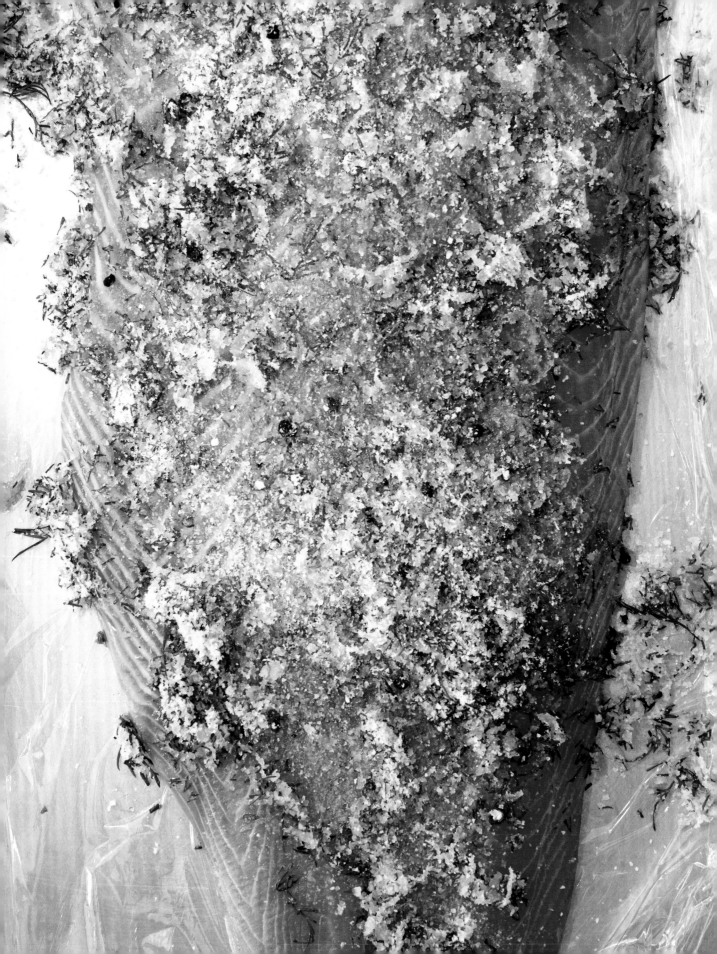

THC
15 mg per serving;
121.8 mg total recipe

Gravlax

Josh Pollack/Rosenberg's Bagels & Delicatessen
Yield: 8 servings; 1¾ pounds

1½ cups kosher salt

1 cup packed fresh dill leaves, plus more for serving

¾ cup granulated sugar

2 tablespoons black peppercorns, lightly crushed

1 tablespoon ground mace

Grated zest of 3 lemons, plus 1 lemon, thinly sliced crosswise

One 2-pound piece center-cut, skin-on salmon fillet (pin bones removed)

3 tablespoons Everclear cannabis tincture (see page 80)

Going viral on the internet is a double-edged sword. Like, maybe, one 4/20, you post a video of yourself making "ganja gravlax," the internet loses its mind, and the health department shows up at your bagel shop to tell you to knock it off. Not that Josh Pollack, who gave us this salmon recipe that he definitely *doesn't* serve at Rosenberg's Bagels & Delicatessen in Denver, would know anything about that. What he does know, however, is that a few tablespoons of strong Everclear-based weed tincture added during gravlax making when you would normally add aquavit makes brunch a lot more interesting. This is a three-day waiting game, so plan ahead. Serve this heady gravlax with bagels and your favorite schmears and vegetables.

In a small bowl, stir together the salt, dill leaves, sugar, peppercorns, mace, and lemon zest, mixing well.

Lay a double-thick sheet of plastic wrap large enough to wrap the salmon on a work surface.

Place the salmon, skin-side down, on the center of the plastic wrap. Season the flesh side evenly with the salt mixture, then sprinkle evenly with the tincture. Wrap the salmon tightly in the plastic wrap and place, flesh-side down, in a baking dish. Refrigerate for 48 hours.

Remove the baking dish from the refrigerator, flip the salmon, and gently massage it, still wrapped, to redistribute the brine. Return to the refrigerator to cure for 24 hours longer. When fully cured, the gravlax will be firm to the touch at the thickest part.

Set a wire rack in a small sheet pan or have ready a clean baking dish.

Unwrap the salmon, discarding any excess brine. Rinse the fish lightly under cool running water and pat dry with paper towels. Place the salmon, skin-side down, on the rack or in the dish and refrigerate, uncovered, overnight.

Cut the salmon against the grain into paper-thin slices to serve.

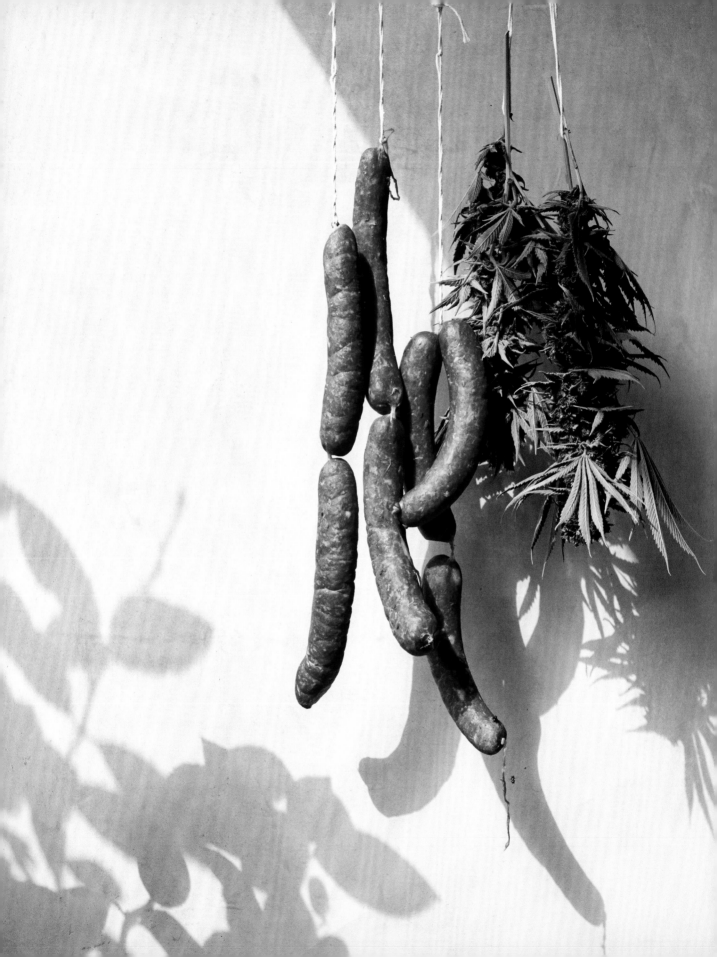

THC
8.8 mg per ¼ pound,
212 mg total recipe

Pot Pepperoni

Justin Severino

Yield: 6 pounds

10 pounds boneless pork shoulder (Boston butt)

4 grams Bactoferm F-RM-52 meat starter culture

½ cup tepid water

½ cup kosher salt

¼ cup granulated sugar

¼ cup smoked paprika

2 teaspoons cayenne pepper

1 tablespoon fennel seeds

1½ teaspoons curing salt #2 (aka Prague powder #2)

1 teaspoon ground allspice

6 tablespoons red wine

5 tablespoons Everclear cannabis tincture (see page 80)

30 feet 46mm hog casings, rinsed to remove salt, then soaked in room-temperature water for 45 to 60 minutes, until pliable

Pittsburgh chef and whole-animal butcher Justin Severino knows his way around meat—and isn't unfamiliar with cannabis either. We tasked him with coming up with a way to combine the two, and this pot-laced pepperoni is the result. Sure, it's ambitious. But it's also amazing. Drop slices on the French Bread Pizza on page 110, or set it out with a plate of the Homemade Ricotta Cheese on page 233 for the kind of cheese-and-charcuterie platter stoner dreams are made of.

Cut the pork into ¾- to 1-inch pieces, pile it into a big container, and put it in the freezer until firm but not frozen, about 30 minutes.

Meanwhile, set up your meat grinder and fit it with the medium die.

Pass half of the chilled meat through the grinder, capturing it in a large bowl. Switch out the medium die for the fine die and pass the remaining meat through the grinder, capturing it in the same bowl.

In a small plastic container, dissolve the starter culture in the water and let stand for 5 minutes.

Meanwhile, add the kosher salt, sugar, paprika, cayenne, fennel seeds, curing salt, allspice, wine, and tincture to the pork and, using your hands, mix until all of the ingredients are evenly distributed. Transfer the sausage to a stand mixer fitted with the paddle attachment. On low speed, add the starter culture solution in a thin stream and continue to mix until the mixture becomes tacky and starts to stick to the sides of the bowl.

Set up your sausage stuffer. Moisten the nozzle of the stuffer with water and slide the casings onto the nozzle. Turn on the stuffer and press some of the meat into the stuffer hopper until about 1 inch of meat protrudes from the tip. Turn off the machine, pull some of the casing from the nozzle over the meat, and tie a knot at the tip, taking care to press out any air pockets. You can use a pin or cake tester to poke any small holes in the casing to release air. Turn the machine

continued

Pot Pepperoni, *continued*

back on and gently press the meat through the stuffer and into the casing, coiling the sausage on your work surface as you work, until you have used up all of the meat.

Cut off any excess casing, pressing out air pockets, and tie a knot at the end. To form the filled casing into links, starting at a tied end, measure off two 12-inch lengths, then twist about four times in one direction between the first and second lengths and twist about four times in the opposite direction after the second length. Repeat until you have a chain of 12-inch-long sausages.

Tie the sausages into loops and load them onto wooden rods on a drying rack. Ferment at 100°F and 100 percent humidity for 12 hours, until the sausages have a pH reading of 4.5 to 5.0. Transfer them to a drying chamber and age at 55°F and 60 percent humidity for 4 weeks, until the pepperoni have lost 30 percent of their original weight or have reached an aw (water activity) reading of 0.84.

Refrigerate the pepperoni for up to 3 months.

THC
10 mg per patty/link;
150 mg total recipe

Hot or Sweet Italian Sausage

Cara Nicoletti

Yield: Fifteen ⅓-pound patties or links

5 pounds ground pork shoulder, very cold

Hot Sausage

¼ cup kosher salt

⅓ cup smoked paprika

4 garlic cloves, mashed to a paste

2 tablespoons fennel seeds, toasted; two-thirds ground to a powder and one-third left whole

4 teaspoons red pepper flakes

2 teaspoons cayenne pepper

1½ teaspoons granulated sugar

1 teaspoon freshly ground black pepper

1 teaspoon coriander seeds

1.9 grams cannabis flower, ground and decarboxylated (see page 55)

¼ cup red wine, chilled

If we were going to ask anyone to show us how to make weed sausage, it had to be Cara Nicoletti, a fourth-generation butcher and baker (and host of MUNCHIES' *Hangover Show*) whose Instagram is basically a shiny rainbow of sausage. Sausage making takes practice to get right—your own personal sausage Instagram might have to delay its launch until you perfect your sausage skills—but it's worth it. Where else are you going to find sausage that gets you high?

Place the pork in the bowl of a stand mixer fitted with the paddle attachment. Turn the mixer to its lowest speed.

To make the hot sausage: Add the salt, paprika, garlic, fennel seeds, red pepper flakes, cayenne, sugar, black pepper, coriander seeds, and cannabis flower to the mixer and mix for exactly 1½ minutes (set a timer!). Add the wine and mix for exactly 1½ minutes. The mixture is now ready to shape into patties or links.

To make the sweet sausage: Add the salt, garlic, fennel seeds, sugar, black pepper, and cannabis flower to the mixer and mix for exactly 1 minute (set a timer!). Add the parsley and rosemary and mix for exactly 1 minute longer. Finally, add the wine and mix for exactly 1 minute. The mixture is now ready to shape into patties or links.

To form sausage patties, divide the mixture into ½-cup portions and flatten into disks about ¾ inch thick. To store in the refrigerator, stack the patties, separating them with squares of parchment paper, then slip into ziplock bags or other airtight containers and refrigerate for up to 5 days. To store in the freezer, arrange the patties in a single layer on parchment paper–lined sheet pans, place in the freezer until frozen, then transfer to ziplock freezer bags and return to the freezer for up to 3 months.

continued

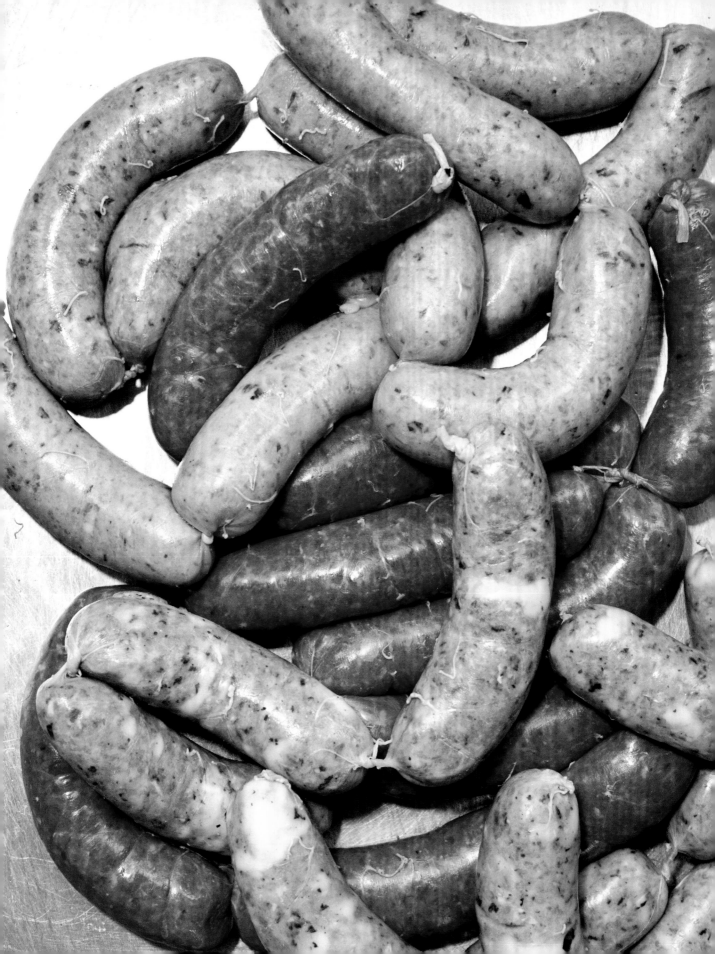

Hot or Sweet Italian Sausage, *continued*

Sweet Sausage

¼ cup kosher salt

3 garlic cloves, mashed to
a paste

2 tablespoons fennel seeds,
toasted; two-thirds ground to a
powder and one-third left whole

1½ teaspoons granulated sugar

1 teaspoon freshly ground
black pepper

1.9 grams cannabis flower,
ground and decarboxylated
(see page 55)

Leaves from 1 large bunch flat-
leaf parsley, finely chopped

Leaves from 4 rosemary sprigs,
finely chopped

½ cup dry white wine, chilled

8 feet 32–36mm hog casings,
rinsed to remove salt, then
soaked in room-temperature
water for 45 to 60 minutes, until
pliable

To form sausage links, set up your sausage stuffer. Moisten the nozzle of the stuffer with water and slide the casings onto the nozzle. Turn on the stuffer and press some of the meat into the stuffer hopper until about 1 inch of meat protrudes from the tip. Turn off the machine, pull some of the casing from the nozzle over the meat, and tie a knot at the tip, taking care to press out any air pockets. You can use a pin or cake tester to poke any small holes in the casing to release air. Turn the machine back on and gently press the meat through the stuffer and into the casing, creating 4-foot lengths. Cut off any excess casing, pressing out air pockets, and tie a knot at the end. Coil the sausage on your work surface as you work, until you have used up all of the meat.

Starting at one tied end, pinch the filled casing into 5-inch lengths, twisting each link a few times in one direction at each pinch. Poke them all over with a pin or toothpick and refrigerate overnight, uncovered, before cooking. To store in the refrigerator, transfer to a ziplock bag in a single layer and refrigerate for up to 5 days. To store in the freezer, arrange the sausages in a single layer on parchment paper–lined sheet pans, place in the freezer until frozen, then transfer to ziplock freezer bags and freeze for up to 3 months.

When ready to cook, heat the oven to 350°F. Place the sausages on a baking sheet and bake until golden and a thermometer inserted reaches 160°F, 17 to 20 minutes.

THC
10 mg per patty/link;
180 mg total recipe

Broccoli Rabe and Provolone Sausage

Cara Nicoletti

Yield: Eighteen ⅓-pound patties or links

1 pound broccoli rabe, tough stem ends discarded

5 pounds ground pork shoulder, very cold

¼ cup kosher salt

7 garlic cloves, mashed to a paste

Grated zest of 1 lemon

4 teaspoons red pepper flakes

1 tablespoon granulated sugar

1 teaspoon freshly ground black pepper

2.8 grams cannabis flower, ground and decarboxylated (see page 55)

1 tablespoon red wine vinegar

¼ cup ice-cold water

1 pound provolone cheese, cut into ¼-inch cubes

9 feet 32–36mm hog casings, rinsed to remove salt, then soaked in room-temperature water for 45 to 60 minutes, until pliable

These cheesy green sausages are especially good grilled and served with a side of peppers and onions. The cheese makes them particularly juicy, so beware when biting in.

Bring a medium saucepan of water to a boil. Meanwhile, fill a large bowl with water and ice.

When the water is boiling, add the broccoli rabe and cook, uncovered, until tender, about 5 minutes. Drain the broccoli rabe and plunge it into the ice water to stop the cooking. Once it has cooled, drain well, then wring thoroughly to remove any water.

Transfer the broccoli rabe to a food processor and process until it is almost paste-like. (You can add a little olive oil to the processor if needed for the blade to move freely.)

Place the pork in the bowl of a stand mixer fitted with the paddle attachment. Turn the mixer to its lowest speed; add the salt, garlic, and lemon zest; and mix for 10 seconds. Add the red pepper flakes, sugar, black pepper, and cannabis flower and mix for exactly 1 minute (set a timer!). Add the broccoli rabe and mix for exactly 1 minute longer. Stir the vinegar into the ice-cold water, add to the mixture, and mix for exactly 30 seconds. Add the cheese and mix for exactly 30 seconds longer. The mixture is now ready to shape into patties or links.

To form sausage patties, divide the mixture into ½-cup portions and flatten into disks about ¾ inch thick. To store in the refrigerator, stack the patties, separating them with squares of parchment paper, then slip into ziplock bags or other airtight containers and refrigerate for up to 5 days. To store in the freezer, arrange the patties in a single layer on parchment paper–lined sheet pans, place in the freezer until frozen, then transfer to ziplock freezer bags and freeze for up to 3 months.

To form sausage links, set up your sausage stuffer. Moisten the nozzle of the stuffer with water and slide the casings onto the nozzle. Turn on the stuffer and press some of the meat into the stuffer hopper until about 1 inch of meat protrudes from the tip. Turn off the machine, pull some of the casing from the nozzle over the meat, and tie a knot at the tip, taking care to press out any air pockets. You can use a pin or cake tester to poke any small holes in the casing to release air. Turn the machine back on and gently press the meat through the stuffer and into the casing, creating 4-foot lengths. Cut off any excess casing, pressing out air pockets, and tie a knot at the end. Coil the sausage on your work surface as you work, until you have used up all of the meat.

Starting at one tied end, pinch the filled casing into 5-inch lengths, twisting each link a few times in one direction at each pinch. Poke them all over with a pin or toothpick and refrigerate overnight, uncovered, before cooking. To store in the refrigerator, transfer to a ziplock bag in a single layer and refrigerate for up to 5 days. To store in the freezer, arrange the sausages in a single layer on parchment paper–lined sheet pans, place in the freezer until frozen, then transfer to ziplock freezer bags and freeze for up to 3 months.

When ready to cook, heat the oven to 350°F. Place the sausages on a baking sheet and bake until golden and a thermometer inserted reaches 160°F, 17 to 20 minutes.

Resources

What you'll be able to get depends, of course, on where you live. But assuming you have some choice in the matter, we've listed out a couple suggestions for how to pair the strains you're most likely to come across as well as some of our favorite pantry providers.

Ry's Pairing Suggestions for Popular Strains

AK-47 • Piney, fruity, sharp • Has a pungent herbal component similar to rosemary; great for chicken.

Blue Dream • Floral, herbal, sweet • This herb-forward varietal is soft enough to use in desserts, but also works well in light, savory dishes.

Bubba Kush • Earthy, sweet, rich • One of the richest-tasting varieties around; its leathery chocolate funk has Scotch-like qualities.

Chemdog • Sharp, funky, gassy • The acridity makes it difficult to pair with most food, but it's good for cutting through fatty foods or adding deep flavor to beverages.

Cookies • Sweet, earthy, rich • Similar chocolate and coffee notes to Gorilla Glue, but sweeter and less obtrusive.

Dosidos • Earthy, sweet, floral • Its sweet, hashy, chocolate-kissed qualities do well in not-too-sweet desserts.

Gorilla Glue • Rich, earthy, gassy • Works well in chocolate desserts or in richer savory dishes.

Green Crack • Tangy, sweet, fruity • A versatile variety with lots of fruity notes; adds a great aromatic component to cocktails and works really well in desserts.

Maui Wowie • Piney, floral, earthy • Works well across most courses.

OG Kush • Sharp, earthy, gassy • Works well with stronger flavors—think coffee, or savory mains like short ribs or lamb.

Purple Urkle • Sweet, floral, fruity • Complex and extremely fragrant, best used for lighter dishes where its uniqueness can shine through.

Sour Diesel • Sharp, bright, gassy • Not quite as acrid and savory as its sister strain Chemdog; it's brighter and plays nicely with fish and chicken.

Strawberry Banana • Fruity, creamy, sweet • Has a delicate, distinct strawberry-banana-smoothie flavor and would work well in something neutral, like cheesecake.

Super Lemon Haze • Sweet, creamy, fruity • Distinct-tasting but lighter, and good for desserts and beverages.

Super Silver Haze • Bright, herbal, floral • Often carries lemongrass and eucalyptus qualities, which go super-well with Thai curry.

Tangie • Citrusy, tangy, floral • An excellent aromatic; adds an incredible, almost-uncanny citrus punch to beverages and sauces.

Pantry Providers

Cannabis Flowers

Most of the recipes in this book are formulated for flower; while it lacks the technical case of concentrates and distillates, it is still our top choice for a holistic cannabis experience. These particular purveyors are some of Southern California's finest.

AJ Sour Diesel: *AJ Sour Diesel*

DNA Genetics: *Kosher Dawg, Lemon Draiz, Strawberry Bubblegum*

IC Collective: *Chem 91, Chem Scout, Diablo OG, T.I.T.S*

Team Elite Genetics: *Candy Nova, Grandma's Cookies, J-1, Tangie*

Top Dawg: *Nigerian Haze*

Urbols: *Jedi OG, Skywalker OG, White Girl*

Vegan Buddha: *Hawaiian Lights*

Wonderbrett: *Candyland, OG9, Orange Banana, OZ Kush, Pineapple OG, Strawberry Bubblegum, Tangieland.*

Concentrates

Solvent-extracted concentrates work well in hot food, because they melt quickly and you only need a little to impart a lot of potency, so the food's flavor can shine through. Terpene-richer concentrates like live resin can add an interesting cannabis note to anything; but watch the heat, as the terpenes will quickly degrade and can impart off flavors.

Beezle Brands: *Bergamot Orange, GG4, Lemon G*

Dabbilicious Extracts: *Banangie OG, Cookies and Cream, Ghost OG, Strawberry OG*

Fresh Off The Bud: *Double OG Sauce*

Harmony Extracts: *Lemon G Sauce, Papaya Nectar Sauce, Mars OG*

Hashy Larry: *Airhead, Forum Cookies, Headband x Lemon Chem, Sweatband*

LoudPack Extracts: *24K, Strawberry Banana*

Quality Concentrates: *XJ-13*

West Coast Cure: *Hardcore OG Sugar*

Culinary Ingredients

These premade culinary ingredients are super-easy if you're unsure about dosing. Just break off 10 milligrams of chocolate and stir into hot milk for delicious hot chocolate, or drizzle 5 milligrams of THC olive oil into a salad dressing.

Binske: *THC Infused Olive Oil (Olio Nuvo, Chipotle, Garlic, Lemon), THC Infused Honey (Wildflower, Yampa Valley, Orange Blossom, Clover), THC Infused Chocolate, THC Infused Chocolate*

Honey Pot: *CBD Honey, Indica (THC) Honey*

Pot d'Huile: *THC Olive Oil*

Distillate/Isolate

Using already-activated distillates makes it incredibly easy to dose edibles, with no guesswork or conversion math necessary. If you know that a particular THC distillate is 92 percent THC, you'll know that 0.1 gram will give you exactly 92 milligrams of THC, and can go from there. THCA crystalline is generally used for smoking, but you can also use it as-is in edibles for a dose of the non-psychoactive (but deeply therapeutic) compound.

Clear Concentrates: *Clear CBD Distillate, Clear THC Distillate*

Elite California: *Elite CBD Distillate*

Higher Vision: *CBD Distillate, THC Distillate*

Rosin

Like solvent concentrates, rosin melts easily into any hot preparation and usually imparts a lot of flavor.

Baroni: *24K, Kosher Dawg, Tangie*

IC Collective: *Chem 91, T.I.T.S*

Team Elite Genetics: *Candy Nova, J-1, Tangie*

Traditional Hash

With their rich, earthy aromas and malleable texture, traditional hash methods, such as temple balls, are incredible for steeping into beverages such as traditional Indian bhang. If the hash is more dry, like traditional Moroccan style blonde hash, it is amazing for grating and can be used in similar ways to kief.

Frenchy Cannoli: *Black Lime Reserve VSOP, Lime Pop VSOP, Orange Turbo VSOP*

Terpenes

Terpenes are essential oils, so they can be used much like other herbal extracts; but they're generally very strong, so start slow and taste, taste, taste. You probably won't want more than a couple drops maximum. Don't expose terpenes to too much heat, as their scents will degrade and change quickly when temperatures climb above 100°F.

Blue River: *GDP, Sour Diesel*

Concentrate Supply Co: *Green Crack, Raz Kush*

Higher Vision: *Blueberry Muffin, Kilimanjaro Cherry, Lemon Jack*

Water-Soluble

Water-soluble formulations are most commonly available as powders, but can also be in a liquid dropper form. THC distillate is normally an oil and thus is not water-soluble, but through modern technology, cannabis-edible wizards are able to shrink THC or CBD particles so they dissolve in water, effectively making them "water soluble." If you can get your hands on water-soluble formulations, you can add them to just about anything that contains liquid.

Cannabinoid Water: *Cannabiplex CBD Nanoparticles*

Concentrate Supply Co: *THC Nanoparticles*

Stillwater Brands: *Ripple Pure 10 THC Powder*

Acknowledgments

Special thanks to the writer of this book, Elise McDonough, for her off- and on-set assistance. Her cannabis knowledge and styling skills, plus her endless supply of weed puns, were invaluable throughout the project. A big thank-you to our publisher, Ten Speed Press, and the dedicated editorial team guiding this project: editor Emily Timberlake, Doug Ogan, Serena Sigona, Carey Jones, designer Kara Plikaitis, and Sharon Silva. As well as the entire staff at Ten Speed, especially Aaron Wehner, Maya Mavjee, Hannah Rahill, Windy Dorresteyn, David Hawk, Daniel Wikey, and Allison Renzulli.

A very special thanks to producer Jason Pinsky, and *Bong Appétit* cast members Vanessa Lavorato and Ry Prichard; first for how their creativity and knowledge has expanded the boundaries of what we know about cannabis cuisine, and also for their extensive help on this book.

Thanks to MUNCHIES publisher John Martin, channel manager Tommy Lucente, Nyasha Shani Foy, and Leslie Stern for their continuous support in our printed efforts. Thanks so much to *Bong Appétit* executive producers Lauren Cynamon and Chris Grosso, co-executive producer Ari Fishman, and the entire cast and crew of *Bong Appétit* involved in making the MUNCHIES Digital and VICELAND series: Gayle Gilman, Erica Winograd, Tracy Wares, David Bienenstock, Elana Schulman, Peter Courtien, Abdullah Saeed, Jason Pinsky, Tami Alfasi, Ariel Algus, Jessica Bahr, Kathleen Flood, Talin Middleton, Carrie Cheek, Allie Stefan, Davina Dobrovech, Armen Karapetian, Hunter Johnson, JonPaul Douglas, Kyle Marchant, Travis Wood, Ronnie Silva, Lex Sadasivan, Alex Wills, Lex Sadasivan, Genéa Gaudet, Ronnie Silva, David Croom, Adam Daroff, Meryl Goodwin, Marley Lister, Katherine Bernard, Arkie Tadesse, Joshua Argue, Will Nails, Zachary Rockwood, Kazmo Kida, Jen White, Ryan Sak, Joeshua Wright, Andre Evans, Robbie Renfrow, Shane Tilston, Sunny Sawhney, George Olivo, Austin Higgins, Karlos Miguel, Dee Wasielewska, and Kalid Hussein.

Thank you to our friends at FremantleMedia, especially Keith Hindle and Elena Magula, and the Tiny Riot team: Regina Leckel, Devon Dunlap, Jessica Porper, and Nathan Rea.

Thank you so much to our agents at the Gernert Company: Anna Worrall, Chris Parris-Lamb, David Gernert, and Paula Breen.

Thanks so much to photographer Marcus Nilsson and world-class photo assistant and hand model, Peter Baker. WE LOVE LA! WE LOVE IT! Thank you to illustrator Ho-Mui Wong for creating beautiful, instructional images that will prevent people from sending themselves to the hospital.

A special thanks to the cutting-edge science used by cannabis lab The Werc Shop and Dr. Jeffrey Raber for helping us understand the test results and efficiency of THC infusions. Science is a powerful drug.

Thanks to marijuana grower Kyle Kushman for providing the marijuana strains Forbidden Fruit, Candyland, and Starberry and Platinum GSC cannabis and Veganic kief for the recipe testing and photography in the book. Thanks to Addison DeMoura and Alex "Poof" from Rezn Extracts, for providing high-end hash and also a Mothership. Special thanks to Purple Frost Genetics for the pre-rolls and flowers, and Kenny Morrow for commenting on the significance of terpenes and extraction technology.

Thanks to our prop stylist, Amy Chin, and her incredible assistant, Lux Wright. Thank you to our recipe testers, Yewande Komolafe and Julie Beth Tanous—we will never look at flies or shortbread cookies the same way ever again. A big thanks to our kitchen interns Andrew Richmond, Justin Ayoub, Widza Gustin, and Alex Burris for helping us during this cookbook process. Special thanks to Yolande Mabiko for truly helping us make this book in ways we could never imagine.

A huge thanks to our dear friend Khuong Phan. Special thanks to Ariel Stark-Benz of Mister Green for providing so many of the beautiful props in this book, along with Little Garage Shop, Stonedware, Concrete Cat, and Group Partner.

None of this would have been possible without the participation of the chefs and collaborators featured, including Aurora Leveroni, Barbara Leung, Bryant Terry, Cara Nicoletti, Chris Lanter, Christine Ha, Courtney McBroom, Dan Nelson, Daniela Soto-Innes, David Posey, David Wilcox, Deuki Hong, Devon Tarby, Don Lee, Erika Nakamura, Fatima Ali, Frank Pinello, Holden Jagger, Iliana Regan, Jasmine Shimoda, Joan Nathan, Jocelyn Guest, John Clark, Jonathan Brooks, Josh Pollack, Justin Severino, Kelly Fields, Louis Tikaram, Mason Hereford, Melissa D'Elia, Melissa Fernandez, Michelle Gayer, Mindy Segal, Natalia Pereira, Rebecca Merhej, Sam Smith, Sarah Kramer, Sheldon Simeon, Thu Tran, Tim Milojevich, Timothy Hollingsworth, Tracy Obolsky, Yoya Takahashi, and Zoe Taylor.

Additional thanks to Colleen Cleary and Joey Lozada at OXO, Barry Frish, Omar Midence, Jason Favreau, Daniel Bonomo, and David DiNoble.

Thanks to VICE co-founders Shane Smith and Suroosh Alvi, co-presidents Andrew Creighton and James Schwab, and the entire VICE team.

The MUNCHIES team would like to thank our former editor in chief, Helen Hollyman, for all her work on this cookbook and art direction on the photo shoot. Thank you to our culinary director, Farideh Sadeghin, for spearheading the recipes in this book, managing our team of recipe testers, and styling the beautiful food; while our editor in chief, Rupa Bhattacharya, smoothed out all the edges and herded all the cats. Massive thanks and gratitude to the entire MUNCHIES family around the globe, and especially our inimitable senior editor Hilary Pollack and wonderful social editor Sydney Mondry, for holding down the fort while we got this book done, as well as staff writer Mayukh Sen and editorial assistant Danielle Wayda, for tolerating endless weed conversations in Slack.

#420blazeit

Index

A

Aioli, 133–34
Ali, Fatima, 100
appetizers
    Blackened Shrimp Cocktail, 113
    Cocktail Sauce, 113
    Coconut Crab Gratin, 114
    Dipping Sauce, 105, 107–8
    French Bread Pizza, 110
    Fried Spring Rolls, 105, 107
    Goat Cheese Sauce, 100
    Pork Wontons, 108–9
    Red Beet Pakoras, 100
    Sour Cream and Onion Nachos, 99
    Sweet Potato Skins with Pancetta
      and Chipotle Crema, 103–4
Apple Bong, 94
Artichoke Dip Risotto, Spinach
    and, 150

B

bacon
    BLAT salad, 123
    Coconut Bacon, 125
    Sweet Potato Skins with Pancetta
      and Chipotle Crema, 103–4
baking mats, silicone, 11, 13
Bananas Foster, 206
Bean Salsa, Sea, 158, 160
beef
    Braised Short Ribs, 158, 160
    Rib-Eye with Weed Chimichurri,
      157
Beet Pakoras, Red, 100
BHO (butane hash oil), 21
Bong Appétit (TV series), 8–9, 14
breads and rolls
    Corn Biscuits, 226
    Dinner Rolls, 224–25
    Herb Focaccia, 223
Broccoli Rabe and Provolone
    Sausage, 244–45
Broccoli Salad, North African, 127
budder texture, 21
butter
    Brown Butter, 141–42
    Brown Butter Gnocchi, 141–42

Buttercream, 211–15
Weed-Infused Brown Butter, 70
Weed-Infused Butter, 68–69

C

cabbage
    Cannabis Kimchi, 234–35
    Coleslaw, 135, 137
cannabinoids, 34–35
cannabis
    acrid, 46
    with alcohol, 38
    antidotes for being too high, 38–39
    citrusy, 48
    cloned, 27
    concentrates and extracts, 21–23,
      28, 34
    dosing, 36–41
    earthy, 48
    fan leaves, 16–17
    flavors, 43–51
    floral, 48
    flower, 14–16, 23
    fruity, 49
    grinding, 11
    herbal, 49
    history of use, 8
    indoor- vs. outdoor-grown, 30
    kief, 16, 18, 23, 28, 53–54
    organic, 30
    pairing food with, 45–46
    potency (THC content), 14–16, 18,
      23, 32, 34, 43 (*see also* dosing)
    quality, 27–29
    sativa vs. indica, 25–26
    from seed, 27
    shopping for, 25–30
    smell, 44
    storing, 28, 30
    strains, 26–27
    sweet, 49
    terpenes, 23, 26, 43–44, 49–51
    trichomes, 17–18
    trim (sugar leaf), 15–16, 23, 28
    water hash, 19–21
    See also tips/techniques for
      preparing weed

cannabis lab, 32–35
cannabis leaves
    Cannabis Leaf Chips, 220
    Cannabis Leaf Pesto, 219
canning jars, 10
CBD (cannabidiol), 34, 38
CBDA (acidic CBD), 34
CBG (cannabigerol), 34
CBN (cannabinol), 35
cheese
    French Bread Pizza, 110
    Goat Cheese Sauce, 100
    Green Mac and Cheese, 145
    Homemade Ricotta Cheese, 233
    Sweet Potato Skins with Pancetta
      and Chipotle Crema, 103–4
cheesecloth, 10
Cherry Elderberry Jam, 230–31
chicken
    Chicken Rice (Riz a Djaj), 152–53
    Double-Lemon Roast Chicken, 165
    Korean Fried Chicken, 166–67
chickpea flour
    Red Beet Pakoras, 100
chiles. *See* peppers, hot
Chimichurri, 157
chocolate/cocoa
    Brownie Sundae, 195
    Frozen Cocoa Pudding Pops, 192
    Salted Chocolate Chip
      Cookies, 196
    Stoner Candy Bites, 190
    Truffles, 189
cilantro
    Creamy Cilantro Kale Salad with
      Coconut Bacon, 124–25
    Creamy Cilantro Vinaigrette, 125
Clark, John, 127
Cocchi Americano
    White Negroni, 88
Coconut Bacon, 125
coconut milk
    Coconut Crab Gratin, 114
    Coconut Seafood Stew
      (Moqueca), 183
    Weed-Infused Coconut Milk, 71
coffee grinder, 11

Coleslaw, 135, 137
Collard Green Melt, 135, 137
Corn Biscuits, 226
Corral, Valerie Leveroni, 141
Crab Gratin, Coconut, 114
cream, heavy
    Frozen Cocoa Pudding Pops, 192
    Homemade Ricotta Cheese, 233
    Honey Rosemary Ice Cream, 193
    Sour Cream and Onion Nachos, 94
    Strawberry Shortcake Trifle,
        201, 203
    Weed-Infused Cream, 72
    Whipped Cream Filling, 211–15
    Whipped Weed-Infused Cream, 73
    Whipped Weed-Infused Honey or
        Syrup, 74–75
crème fraîche
    Sweet Potato Skins with Pancetta
        and Chipotle Crema, 103–4
Cucumber and Citrus Salad, 119
curry
    Green Shellfish Curry, 180
    Homemade Curry Paste, 181

D
dabbing, 11, 21–23
decarboxylation, 55, 58–59
decarboxylation machine, 13
D'Elia, Melissa, 103, 232
desserts
    Adult Celebration Cake, 211–15
    After-Dinner Mint Gummies,
        208–9
    Bananas Foster, 206
    Brownie Sundae, 195
    Buttercream, 211–15
    Frozen Cocoa Pudding Pops, 192
    Honey Rosemary Ice Cream, 193
    Raspberry and Peach Pie, 198, 200
    Salted Chocolate Chip Cookies,
        196
    Stoner Candy Bites, 190
    Strawberry "Cheesecake," 205
    Strawberry Shortcake Trifle,
        201, 203
    Truffles, 189
    Whipped Cream Filling, 211–15
Dipping Sauce, 105, 107–8
Dirty Martini, 87
distillates, 21, 23
dosing, 36–41

drinks
    Apple Bong, 94
    Dirty Martini, 87
    French 75, 90
    Herbal-Infused Vermouth, 88
    Manhattan, 87
    Margarita, 93
    Sangria, 91
    Simple Syrup, 90
    White Negroni, 88

E
eggs
    Honey Rosemary Ice Cream, 193
    Strawberry Shortcake Trifle,
        201, 203
equipment, 10–13
Everclear, 79
Everclear Cannabis Tincture, 80

F
Fields, Kelly, 192
fish and shellfish
    Blackened Shrimp Cocktail, 113
    Coconut Crab Gratin, 114
    Coconut Seafood Stew
        (Moqueca), 183
    Confit Octopus, 184
    Fried Soft-Shell Crab with
        Shishito Pepper Mole, 177–78
    Gravlax, 237
    Green Shellfish Curry, 180
    Grilled Oysters, 174
    Grilled Whole Sea Bream, 173
    Pakalolo Poke Bowl, 169
    Swordfish Teriyaki, 170
flavors of cannabis, 43–51
fruit
    Cucumber and Citrus Salad, 119
    Sangria, 91
    Summer Tomato and Stone Fruit
        Salad, 120
    See also individual fruits

G
gin
    Dirty Martini, 87
    French 75, 90
    White Negroni, 88
Glycerin Cannabis Tincture, 83
Gnocchi, Brown Butter, 141–42

grapefruit liqueur
    Margarita, 93
grape press, 13
grater, microplane, 10
Gravlax, 237

H
Hà, Christine, 105
Herbal-Infused Vermouth, 88
herb grinder, 11
herbs
    Creamy Cilantro Kale Salad with
        Coconut Bacon, 124–25
    Creamy Cilantro Vinaigrette, 125
    Honey Rosemary Ice Cream, 193
    White Wine and Herb
        Vinaigrette, 120
Hereford, Mason, 135
high-performance liquid
        chromatography (HPLC), 32
Hollingsworth, Tim, 93, 224
honey
    Honey Rosemary Ice Cream, 193
    Roasted Vegetables with Whipped
        Weed-Infused Honey, 130
    Whipped Weed-Infused Honey or
        Syrup, 74–75
Hong, Deuki, 166
Hymanson, Sarah, 119

I
ice cream
    Brownie Sundae, 195
    Honey Rosemary Ice Cream, 193
infusions
    alcohol-based, 77–80
    calculating potency, 39–41
    equipment, 10, 13
    Everclear Cannabis Tincture, 80
    fats, role of, 62
    Glycerin Cannabis Tincture, 83
    Nitrous Green Dragon, 77–78
    Weed-Infused Brown Butter, 70
    Weed-Infused Butter, 68–69
    Weed-Infused Coconut Milk, 71
    Weed-Infused Cream, 72
    Weed-Infused Oil, 64–65
    Whipped Weed-Infused Cream, 73
isolate (extract), 21–22
isopropyl alcohol, 11

J

Jagger, Holden, 234
Jam, Cherry Elderberry, 230–31

K

Kale Salad, Creamy Cilantro, with
    Coconut Bacon, 124–25
ketchup
    Cocktail Sauce, 113
    Russian Dressing, 137
kief shaker, 57
Kim, Beverly, 127
Kimchi, Cannabis, 234–35
Kimchi Ganja Salt, 166–67
Kramer, Sara, 119
Kushman, Kyle, 32

L

Lamb, Yogurt-Marinated, 162
Lanter, Chris, 161
Lavorato, Vanessa, 9
Lee, Don, 77
lemon
    Double-Lemon Roast Chicken, 165
    Preserved Lemons, 228
Leveroni, Aurora, 141
limonene, 50–51
linalool, 51

M

Mac and Cheese, Green, 145
Manhattan, 83
Margarita, 93
mayonnaise
    Alabama White Sauce, 161
    Russian Dressing, 137
Merhej, Rebecca, 152
mezcal
    Apple Bong, 94
    Nitrous Green Dragon, 77–78
milk
    Frozen Cocoa Pudding Pops, 192
    Homemade Ricotta Cheese, 233
    Honey Rosemary Ice Cream, 193
mirin
    Homemade Teriyaki Sauce, 170
Mushrooms, Fried Mixed, 133–34
myrcene, 51

N

Nachos, Sour Cream and Onion, 94
Nakamura, Erika, 162
Nathan, Joan, 165, 228

Nelson, Daniel, 88
Nicoletti, Cara, 241, 244
Nitrous Green Dragon, 77–78
Nom Wah Tea Parlor (Chinatown,
    NYC), 108

O

Oil, Weed-Infused, 64–65
onions
    Sour Cream and Onion Nachos, 94
orange liqueur
    Sangria, 91
oranges
    Cucumber and Citrus Salad, 119

P

Pancetta and Chipotle Crema, Sweet
    Potato Skins with, 103–4
parchment paper, 11
pasta & grains
    Brown Butter Gnocchi, 141–42
    Chicken Rice (Riz a Djaj), 152–53
    Green Mac and Cheese, 145
    Peanut Butter Noodles, 146
    Polenta, 158, 160
    Sausage Pappardelle Bolognese,
        149
    Spinach and Artichoke Dip
        Risotto, 150
peaches
    Raspberry and Peach Pie, 198, 200
    Summer Tomato and Stone Fruit
        Salad, 120
peanuts/peanut butter
    Homemade Peanut Butter, 232
    Peanut Butter Noodles, 146
    Peanut Butter Sauce, 195
pellet smoker, 13
peppers, hot
    Fried Soft-Shell Crab with
        Shishito Pepper Mole, 177–78
    Homemade Curry Paste, 181
    Sweet Potato Skins with Pancetta
        and Chipotle Crema, 103–4
Pinello, Frank, 233
pinene, 51
Pizza, French Bread, 110
Polenta, 158, 160
Pollack, Josh, 237
pork
    Broccoli Rabe and Provolone
        Sausage, 244–45

Hot or Sweet Italian Sausage,
    241, 243
    Pork Wontons, 108–9
    Pot Pepperoni, 239–40
    Sausage Pappardelle Bolognese, 149
    "Sugaree" Pork Ribs, 161
    See also bacon
Posey, Anna, 208
potato chips
    Sour Cream and Onion Nachos, 94
    Stoner Candy Bites, 190
potatoes
    Brown Butter Gnocchi, 141–42
    Hasselback Potatoes, 129
Prichard, Ry, 9, 39, 45, 62
projects
    Broccoli Rabe and Provolone
        Sausage, 244–45
    Cannabis Kimchi, 234–35
    Cannabis Leaf Chips, 220
    Cannabis Leaf Pesto, 219
    Cherry Elderberry Jam, 230–31
    Corn Biscuits, 226
    Dinner Rolls, 224–25
    Gravlax, 237
    Herb Focaccia, 223
    Homemade Peanut Butter, 232
    Homemade Ricotta Cheese, 233
    Hot or Sweet Italian Sausage,
        241, 243
    Pot Pepperoni, 239–40
    Preserved Lemons, 228
The Publican (Chicago), 158

R

Raber, Jeff, 32, 34
Ras el Hanout Vinaigrette, 127
Raspberry and Peach Pie, 198, 200
resin, live, 22, 44
Rice, Chicken (Riz a Djaj), 152–53
Risotto, Spinach and Artichoke Dip,
    150
rosin, 22
Russo, Ethan, 44

S

sake
    Homemade Teriyaki Sauce, 170
salad dressings
    Creamy Cilantro Vinaigrette, 125
    Ras el Hanout Vinaigrette, 127
    Russian Dressing, 137

White Wine and Herb
Vinaigrette, 120
salads & vegetables
BLAT salad, 123
Coleslaw, 135, 137
Collard Green Melt, 135, 137
Creamy Cilantro Kale Salad with
Coconut Bacon, 124–25
Cucumber and Citrus Salad, 119
Fried Mixed Mushrooms, 133–34
Hasselback Potatoes, 129
North African Broccoli Salad, 127
Roasted Vegetables with Whipped
Weed-Infused Honey, 130
Summer Tomato and Stone Fruit
Salad, 120
Za'atar, 119
Salsa, Sea Bean, 158, 160
sandwiches
Collard Green Melt, 135, 137
Sangria, 91
sauce (extract), 22
sauces
Aioli, 133–34
Alabama White Sauce, 161
Cannabis Leaf Pesto, 219
Chimichurri, 157
Cocktail Sauce, 113
Dipping Sauce, 105, 107–8
Goat Cheese Sauce, 100
Homemade Curry Paste, 181
Homemade Teriyaki Sauce, 170
Peanut Butter Sauce, 195
Sea Bean Salsa, 158, 160
Shishito Pepper Mole, 177–78
Sweet Soy Sauce, 169
sausages
Broccoli Rabe and Provolone
Sausage, 244–45
Hot or Sweet Italian Sausage,
241, 243
Sausage Pappardelle Bolognese,
149
scale, digital kitchen, 10
Severino, Justin, 239
shatter (extract), 22
Shimoda, Jasmine, 124, 205
shrimp. See fish and shellfish
Simeon, Sheldon, 169
Simple Syrup, 90
Apple Bong, 94
Margarita, 93

slow cooker, 13
Smith, Sam, 120
smoke gun, 13
smoking vs. edibles, 37
Soto-Innes, Daniela, 177
Sour Cream and Onion Nachos, 94
sous vide cooking, 58
soy sauce
Homemade Teriyaki Sauce, 170
Sweet Soy Sauce, 169
spatulas, rubber, 10
spice ball, 13
spinach
Green Mac and Cheese, 145
Spinach and Artichoke Dip
Risotto, 150
Spring Rolls, Fried, 105, 107
strainers, mesh, 10
strawberries
Strawberry "Cheesecake," 205
Strawberry Shortcake Trifle,
201, 203
Sweet Potato Skins with Pancetta
and Chipotle Crema, 103–4
syrup
Simple Syrup, 90
Whipped Weed-Infused Honey or
Syrup, 74–75

T
Takahashi, Yoya, 170
Tarby, Devon, 94
Taylor, Zoe, 230
tea strainer, 13
tequila
Margarita, 93
THC (Delta-9-tetrahydrocannabinol)
content/potency, 14–16, 23, 32
decarboxylating, 55, 58–59
dosing, 36–41
in kief, 18
THCA (acidic THC), 17, 35, 39–41
THCV (tetrahydrocannabivarin), 35
thermometer, instant-read, 10
Tikaram, Louis, 180
tips/techniques for preparing weed
decarboxylation, 55, 58–59
drying and curing, 56
kief shaker, 57
making/using kief, 53–54

tomatoes
BLAT salad, 123
French Bread Pizza, 110
Roasted Tomatoes, 178
Summer Tomato and Stone Fruit
Salad, 120
Tran, Thu, 190

U
United States Department of
Agriculture (USDA), 30

V
vermouth
Dirty Martini, 87
Herbal-Infused Vermouth, 88
Manhattan, 83
White Negroni, 88

W
water hash, 19–21
wax texture, 21
Werc Shop, 32
whiskey
Manhattan, 83
White Negroni, 88
Wilcox, David, 173
wine
Sangria, 91
White Wine and Herb
Vinaigrette, 120
Wontons, Pork, 108–9

Y
Yogurt-Marinated Lamb, 162

Z
Za'atar, 119

Copyright © 2018 by Vice Food, LLC.
Illustrations copyright © 2018 by Ho-Mui Wong.

All rights reserved.
Published in the United States by Ten Speed Press,
an imprint of the Crown Publishing Group, a division
of Penguin Random House LLC, New York.

www.crownpublishing.com
www.tenspeed.com

Ten Speed Press and the Ten Speed Press
colophon are registered trademarks of
Penguin Random House LLC.

Library of Congress Cataloging-in-Publication Data

    Names: McDonough, Elise, 1980- editor. | Nilsson, Marcus
(Photographer),
        photographer. | Wong, Ho-Mui, illustrator. | Editors of
Munchies.
    Title: Bong appetit : mastering the art of cooking with
weed / the Editors of
        Munchies with Elise McDonough ; photographs by
Marcus Nilsson ;
        illustrations by Ho-Mui Wong.
    Description: First edition. | California : Ten Speed Press,
2018. | Includes
        bibliographical references and index.
    Identifiers: LCCN 2018011118
    Subjects: LCSH: Cooking (Marijuana) | Snack foods. |
Desserts. | LCGFT:
        Cookbooks.
    Classification: LCC TX819.M25 B66 2018 | DDC
641.6/379—dc23
    LC record available at https://lccn.loc.gov/2018011118

Hardcover ISBN: 978-0-399-58010-9
eBook ISBN: 978-0-399-58011-6

Printed in China

Design by Kara Plikaitis

10 9 8 7 6 5 4 3 2 1

First Edition

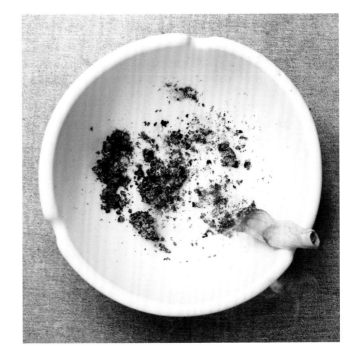